Management of Vitreo-Retinal Disease

Springer
London
Berlin
Heidelberg
New York
Barcelona
Budapest
Hong Kong
Milan
Paris
Santa Clara
Singapore
Tokyo

A.H. Chignell and D. Wong

Management of Vitreo-Retinal Disease

A Surgical Approach

Illustrated by T.R. Tarrant

With 99 Figures
37 in Full Colour

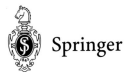

Springer

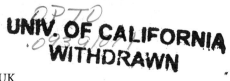
Anthony Chignell, FRCS
St Thomas' Hospital, London, UK

David Wong, FRCS
Royal Liverpool University Hospital, St Paul's Eye Unit,
Prestcott Street, Liverpool L7 8XP, UK

Cover illustrations: Front cover insets: Figure 1.2 (the ora serrata); Figure 17.1 (feathery gas lens opacities); Figure 4.7 (retinal detachment). Back cover inset: Figure 1.4 (the normal fundus).

ISBN 3–540–76082–2 Springer-Verlag Berlin Heidelberg New York

British Library Cataloguing in Publication Data
Chignell, A.H. (Anthony Hugh), 1939–
    Management of vitreo-retinal disease: a surgical approach
    1. Retina – Surgery 2. Vitreous body – Surgery 3. Retina –
    Diseases 4. Vitreous body – Diseases
    I. Title II. Wong, David H.W.
    617.7'35'059
ISBN 3540760822

Library of Congress Cataloging-in-Publication Data
Chignell, A.H.
    Management of vitreo-retinal disease: a surgical approach/A.H.
Chignell and D. Wong.
        p.   cm.
    Includes bibliographical references and index.
    ISBN 3–540–76082–2 (pbk.: alk. paper)
    1. Retinal detachment – Surgery. 2. Proliferative
vitreoretinopathy – Surgery. 3. Vitrectomy. I. Wong, D. (David),
1952– . II. Title.
    [DNLM: 1. Retinal Detachment – surgery. 2. Vitreoretinopathy,
Proliferative – surgery. 3. Vitrectomy. WW 270 C534m 1998]
RE603.C457   1998
617.7'35059 – dc21
DNLM/DLC   98–20113
for Library of Congress   CIP

Typeset by EXPO Holdings, Malaysia
Printed by Kyodo Printing Co. (S'pore) Pte. Ltd., Singapore
28/3830-543210 Printed on acid-free paper

Preface

This book is a short account of conditions that may be treated by vitreo-retinal surgery. It is intended for all levels of junior ophthalmologists to enhance an apprenticeship-based training by assisting in the development of vitreo-retinal surgical skills. Also we hope that senior ophthalmologists will find it useful to update their knowledge and that it may benefit other workers in ophthalmic care such as optometrists and nurse practitioners. We have emphasised the principles of approach and management in an attempt to achieve the desired effect at surgery in the simplest way with the least morbidity. We have not attempted to describe all the various operations and techniques available which will undoubtedly continue to change but have only emphasised those that we favour.

The greater part of the work of the vitreo-retinal surgeon is still the management of rhegmatogenous retinal detachment; the text reflects this work and particularly emphasises the role of examination and surgical planning.

We discuss pars plana vitrectomy which has allowed the treatment of conditions other than that of retinal detachment and this will be an expanding field in the future.

A suggested reading list at the end of the text has been included for those who wish to enhance and extend their knowledge of the topics covered. We are most grateful to the following who have helped us in the preparation of this text:

Illustrations have been provided by Professor John Marshall (Fig. 1.1a and b), Mr Tim Ffytche (Fig. 11.3) and Mr D. Chauhan (Fig.19.5). Mr Don Nelson has helped with some of the artwork and Mr Tom Williamson and Mr Christopher Hammond have read the text and have made numerous helpful suggestions about layout and content. Mrs Maureen Forde and Miss Hazel Hollands have provided unfailing and enthusiastic secretarial support. Lastly, it has been a great pleasure for us to work with Mr Terry Tarrant who has done the greater part of the artwork and whose skills have enormously enhanced the text.

Anthony Chignell and David Wong
1998

Contents

1 Basic Information

This chapter covers basic information on the anatomy and physiology of the retina, vitreous, choroid and sclera that we consider relevant to vitreo-retinal surgery. Anatomical and surgical landmarks are included.

The Retina

Anatomy and Function

The vitreo-retinal surgeon is most often concerned about the effect of disease upon the function of the retina. Function is affected when either the retina detaches causing reduction of peripheral or central vision or, if not detached, central vision is altered by disturbance of the macula. The retina is classically described as having 10 layers: the pigment epithelium, the layer of rods and cones, the external limiting membrane, the outer nuclear layer, the outer plexiform layer, the inner nuclear layer, the inner plexiform layer, the ganglion-cell layer, the nerve-fibre layer and the internal limiting membrane, which is nearest the vitreous cavity (Fig. 1.1a,b).

The retina extends from the optic disc to its anterior extremity, the ora serrata. The macula lutea is so called because of its yellow colour, which is more apparent in post-mortem eyes. The centre of the macula is the fovea, which subserves central vision.

The pigment epithelium is a single layer of cells which contain a variable amount of pigment, and give rise to the mottled appearance of the fundus. There are tight junctions between the cells of the epithelium, which itself forms part of the blood–ocular barrier regulating metabolic exchange between the retina and the choriocapillaris.

The visual cells of the retina are the rods and cones; so called because of the appearance of the outer segments of the cells on light microscopy. On electron microscopy the membranes of the outer segments are elaborated into regular series of lamellae, and make intricate cellular connections with the pigment epithelial cells.

The external limiting membrane separates the cell bodies of the rods and cones from their nuclei. It is formed by the fibres of the Müller's cells, which form part of the cellular architecture of the retina.

The outer nuclear layer is formed by the nuclei of the visual cells, which send fibres to make synaptic connections with dendrites of the bipolar and the horizontal cells in the outer plexiform layer. The inner nuclear layer is formed by the cell bodies of the bipolar cells, which synapse with the ganglion cells at the inner plexiform layer. Convergence of

1

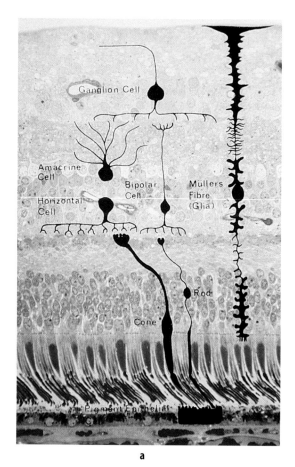

a

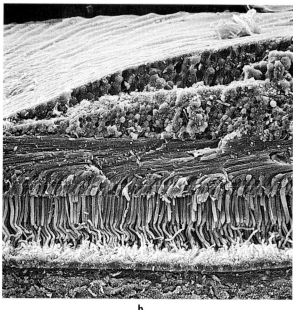

b

Fig. 1.1. a Cross-section of retina to show retinal layers; **b** scanning electron microscope section of retina in the macular region.

neural connections results in each ganglion cell receiving input from a number of photoreceptors. The dendrites from the ganglion cells form the nerve-fibre layer and carry processed information up the optic nerve.

When a retinal detachment involves the macula, its function is impaired and visual acuity is reduced. Diseases of the macula give rise to symptoms of metamorphopsia (distortion), macropsia or micropsia (larger or smaller images) and dyschromatopsia (disturbance of colour). Due to disruption of the cone pigment epithelial relationship by the presence of subretinal fluid, reattachment of a detached macula may result in only partial recovery of visual acuity.

Blood Supply to the Retina

The inner retina derives its blood supply from the retinal blood vessels and the outer retina from the choroid. Detached retina carries with it its own blood supply and can remain viable for many months. The retinal blood vessels do not have any autonomic nerve supply and blood flow is controlled by autoregulation. This mechanism protects the perfusion of the eye against fluctuation in systemic blood pressure and intraocular pressure. As in the brain, the vascular resistance of the blood vessels in the eye increases with a rise in systemic blood pressure, so that blood flow is not affected.

Similarly, a rise in intraocular pressure leads to a reduction in the vascular tone to ensure that blood flow is maintained.

The retinal blood vessels are situated on the inner aspect of the retina with capillaries supplying the inner layers of the retina. They often bleed into the vitreous cavity when retinal tears are caused by vitreous traction.

Peripheral Retina

The peripheral retina includes the ora serrata and the retina between the ora and the equator of the eye. As the majority of retinal breaks and degeneration are found in this part of the retina, it is a region of particular importance to the retinal surgeon and demands painstaking observation and experience in interpretation. Various types of peripheral retinal degenerations and their relevance are described in Chap. 12.

Ora Serrata

The ora serrata is easily seen in the aphakic eye by indirect ophthalmoscopy, but is only seen in the phakic eye when pushed into view with scleral depression. The neuro-epithelium of the retina continues into the pars plana as the non-pigmented epithelium of the pars plana. The dentate processes that make up the ora serrata are most prominent on the nasal side; on the temporal aspect they have a rather flat, inconspicuous appearance, particularly in the lower temporal quadrant. The processes show considerable individual variation and are less obvious in children. It is important to be aware of local anatomical variations of the ora so that physical signs are not misinterpreted and lead to the treatment of harmless conditions. The following important variations in the ora serrata may be found: (Fig. 1.2).

1. Meridional folds are posterior and upward projections of full thickness retina. Occasionally these are associated with small round retinal breaks at the posterior aspect of the fold. A meridional complex is defined as an alignment of the meridional fold and a ciliary process.

2. An enclosed oral bay formed by joined processes. This may be mistaken for a peripheral retinal break.

3. Pars plana cysts are opalescent and usually small.

4. Granular tissue (tags) consists of small, whitish opacities of various shapes and sizes, probably derived from the retina itself. Such opacities are often found in the postoral region, particularly on the nasal side either on the surface of the retina itself or in the vitreous. They may be mistaken for small peripheral opercula; however, their small size, their peripheral distribution and their multiplicity are distinguishing features.

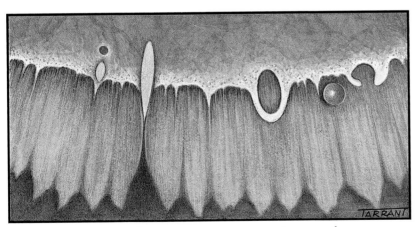

Fig. 1 2. The ora serrata. A meridional fold and retinal hole is seen at **a**; a meridional complex at **b**; an enclosed oral bay at **c**; and a pars plana cyst at **d**.

a b   c d

Embryology of the Retina

The retina is of neuro-ectodermal origin. It is derived embryologically from the optic cup, which is an outgrowth from the forebrain. The optic cup consists of two layers of neuro-ectodermal cells separated by a space. The outer layer of cells eventually forms the retinal pigment epithelium and the inner layer the neuro-sensory retina. It is the potential space between these two layers which reopens in the process of retinal detachment.

Intraretinal Apposition

The rod and cone outer segments form intricate interdigitation with the retinal pigment epithelial cells. Electromicrographs of the retina show the photoreceptor outer segment to form stacks of flattened membranous saccules within the retinal pigment epithelial cell. Although not clearly understood, the forces that tend to keep the retinal layers in apposition include a high choroidal osmotic pressure, hydrostatic forces and an active solute-linked transport system activated by the retinal pigment epithelium. These forces may be augmented by the potential binding effect of the two layers of the retina by the intercellular mucopolysaccharide layer.

The efficiency of these mechanisms is shown by the fact that post-mortem and clinical studies have demonstrated that the majority of retinal breaks exposing the subretinal space to the vitreous cavity do not progress to retinal detachment. The occurrence of rhegmatogenous retinal detachment indicates that the posterior movement of fluid across pigment epithelium has been exceeded by the rate of recruitment of fluid from the vitreous cavity. The more pronounced the vitreous traction upon the retina, the greater will be the chance of a breakdown of the adhesive forces; thus, retinal tears are more likely to proceed to retinal detachment than retinal holes. Also, large breaks allowing easier access for retro-hyaloid fluid to the subretinal space are more likely to lead to detachment than smaller ones.

In spite of the apparent intricate interdigitation of rods and cones outer segments with the retinal pigment epithelium, and in spite of the rupture of these connections during retinal detachment, visual recovery is quickly restored when retinal apposition is re-established after surgery.

Recognising Normal and Detached Retina

The normal retina is transparent. Retinal blood vessels within it are seen, as are those of the underlying choroid. The macula is recognised by the slightly darker appearance of the underlying retinal pigment epithelium but luteal pigmentation is more obvious when the retina is detached. When detached, the retina becomes opalescent and takes on a greyish hue because of intraretinal oedema and the retinal surface can often appear corrugated. The view of the underlying choroidal vasculature is obscured. Shallow posterior retinal detachment is best detected by the slit-lamp biomicroscopy whilst shallowly elevated peripheral retina is best observed using scleral indentation and indirect ophthalmoscopy (Fig. 1.3).

The Vitreous

Ultrastructure

The vitreous humour is a transparent gel like structure occupying the posterior segment of the eye. The major constituents of the vitreous are water, collagen fibrils, glycosaminoglycans, soluble proteins and microfibrils. The collagen is a protein comprised of three polypeptide chains arranged in a triple helix. There are at least 18 known types of collagen and more are being described. Those that make up the vitreous collagen are mainly type II, and type IX. The glycosaminoglycans such as hyaluronic acid are attached to the protein core of the collagen fibrils by non-covalent bonds. It is this interaction of the glycosaminoglycans with the collagen fibrils which gives the vitreous its gel structure.

In a normal young eye, the vitreous is attached to the whole surface of the retina, the optic-nerve head, the pars plana, the ciliary body, and the posterior lens surface. The vitreous base refers to a 4 to 5 mm circumferential zone of enhanced adhesion between the vitreous body and the pars plana, ora serrata and the anterior retina. With indirect ophthalmoscopy, the vitreous base over the retina may be recognised by a light-grey appearance.

In the emmetropic adult eye, the vitreous occupies a volume of approximately 4 ml. The volume varies with the size of the globe and is greatly increased in high myopia (up to 10 ml or more). The dimensions of the collagen fibrils are smaller than the wavelength of the visible spectrum of light, thus when the gel is normal, the vitreous is transparent and can only be observed on the slit-lamp or at the time of vitrectomy by light scatter. It is therefore best seen by maximising the angle between the illumination and the line of observation. In the case of slit-lamp biomicroscopy, a widely dilated pupil is necessary. Even then observing vitreous in the posterior cavity is difficult because the incident light and observation path are almost co-axial. With ageing of the normal vitreous, its gel like structure changes to a more liquid state. The collagen fibrils collapse together and form bundles that are large enough to reflect light and therefore to become more visible.

Embryology of the Vitreous

The vitreous develops in three stages. The first stage occurs between 3 and 6 weeks when the primary vitreous is derived from the inner layer of the optic vesicle, tissue from the lens vesicle, and mesodermal fibrils associated with the hyaloid artery. The primary vitreous persists into adult life and ultimately becomes the hyaloid canal. Persistent and hypoplastic primary vitreous is a rare developmental anomaly which may present in early infancy as leucocoria, vitreous haemorrhage, microphthalmos and glaucoma. The secondary vitreous develops in the second stage (between 3 and 10 weeks) and is derived from the inner neuro-ectoderm of the optic cup. Thus, the vitreous fibres are continuous with the Müller foot plates of the retina. The hyaloid artery system develops up to the 8-week stage and then atrophies in a posterior to anterior direction. This artery may persist after full gestation and may cause retro-lenticular haemorrhage, or be associated with localised lens opacity. The third stage occurs from 10 weeks. The tertiary vitreous consists of fibrils from the ciliary epithelium of the optic cup, which condenses eventually to become the suspensory ligament of the lens. The close relationship between the development of the retina and the vitreous explains, at least in part, the importance of the vitreous in contributing to the pattern of vitreo-retinal surgical disease.

Vitreous Attachments and Detachments

The normal vitreous is closely applied to the inner layers of the retina and is continuous with the internal limiting membrane. It is particularly firmly attached to the retina around the disc, at the macula to superficial retinal vessels, and at the vitreous base, an area that extends for approximately 2 mm on either side of the ora serrata; thus it is firmly attached to the retina posteriorly and to the pars plana anteriorly. The points of firm attachment of the vitreous have an important bearing on the patterns of problems arising as a consequence of vitreous detachment. The posterior part of the vitreous base is of particular importance, for it is here that traction is exerted if detached posterior vitreous swings freely at this point of anchorage. Enhanced adhesions to blood vessels can lead to avulsed loops of vessels and vitreous haemorrhage as a result of vitreous traction. The firm adhesion of the vitreous to the disc and retinal blood vessels determines the configuration of fibrovascular proliferation in diabetic retinopathy.

The mode of vitreous detachment is dealt with in Chap. 3.

Vitreo-retinal Interface

Traditionally it is believed that vitreous gel separates as a body from the retina posteriorly. The so-called posterior face is made of condensed vitreous cortex and the surface of the retina is demarcated by the internal limiting membrane. In most ordinary cases of posterior vitreous detachment, the posterior hyaloid does appear to have separated completely from the internal limiting membrane. However, whether or not there is complete separation of gel, or whether there remains a layer of cortex adherent to the internal limiting lamina, is controversial. In patients where the vitreous cortex appears to be split (vitreoschisis) a layer of cortex remains adherent to the internal limiting lamina. This layer may be identified at the time of vitrectomy. When this residual layer occurs at the macula the intragel cavity is known as the premacular bursar and is seen in posterior retina in cases of proliferative diabetic retinopathy.

There is also evidence that the cleavage plane of posterior vitreous detachment (PVD) can occur at the internal limiting lamina because type IV collagen (a constituent of the internal limiting lamina) has been found in posterior vitreous detachments in post-mortem eyes. In cases of 'sub-hyaloid' haemorrhage from Terson's syndrome or from a macroaneurysm, the blood is located external to the internal limiting lamina.

The attachments of the internal limiting lamina to the Müller foot plates vary in different parts of the retina. At the vitreous base, the collagen fibres are in direct continuity with the Müller foot plates, giving great strength of attachment to the vitreous in this region, thus vitreous detachment does not normally occur at the vitreous base. In peripheral retina, the inner limiting lamina is attached to the Müller cells by specialised tight junctions within the foot plates. At the posterior pole these tight junctions are missing.

It is likely that the plane of vitreo-retinal cleavage of posterior vitreous detachment is determined by the disease process inducing vitreous detachment and that the actual plane of separation is variable.

The Choroid

Anatomy and Function

The choroid is made up mainly of blood vessels and is firmly adherent to the retina. The blood flow through the choroid is high and it has been suggested that this enables it to act as a 'heat sink', offering protection to the retina against thermal damage from light (and lasers) falling onto the retina. The blood flow through the choroid is responsive to metabolic changes and to the concentration of dissolved gases in the blood. Increased concentration of carbon dioxide in the blood, and to a lesser extent decreased concentration of oxygen, causes vasodilatation of the choroidal and retinal blood vessels. Hypocapnia induced by ventilation during general anaesthesia leads to vasoconstriction of the choroid, which is often desirable. Vaso-constriction of the choroid is useful for surgery involving choroidal biopsies, the excision of intra-ocular tumours and choroidal puncture for drainage of subretinal fluid during retinal detachment surgery.

On the external surface of the choroid is a delicate layer of collagen meshwork, the suprachoroidal lamina, which is adherent to the sclera. The supra-choroidal lamina is a potential cleavage plane, and can be split and distended by effusion and blood (e.g. serous choroidal detachment and choroidal haemorrhage). The choroid contains numerous melanocytes and fibroblasts, and appears dark in colour on its external surface. It also contains the long and short posterior ciliary arteries and nerves. The choroidal blood vessels are supported by a stroma of collagen tissue with elastin and reticulin fibres. The arterial supply comes from the short posterior ciliary arteries, which penetrate the sclera around the optic nerve. The venous drainage is organised into lobules and exits from the eye at the equator via the vortex veins. The vortex veins drain the entire choroid, and exit from the eye through an oblique passage through the sclera at the equator of the globe. The ampullae of the vortex veins are dilated trunks formed just before the veins exit the sclera.

The blood vessels on the inner aspect of the choroid are made up of closely packed capillaries (the choriocapillaris). The capillaries of the choroid are fenestrated. These vessels provide nutrition to the outer two-thirds of the neuro-sensory retina, from which it is separated by a basal lamina known as Bruch's membrane.

The choroid extends anteriorly to become the uvea of the pars plana, ciliary processes, ciliary body and iris. Clinically therefore, choroidal detachment extends further anteriorly than the ora serrata, and suprachoroidal blood can track anteriorly into the anterior chamber via the iris root attachment to the scleral spur. Thus choroidal detachments may be drained at the pars plana when sclerotomies are prepared at the beginning of a vitrectomy procedure.

The Sclera

Anatomy

The sclera is constructed of dense collagen fibres running as bands in all directions. In a normal eye it is about 1 mm thick in the posterior part of the globe, but becomes progressively thinner as it approaches the annulus of the rectus muscle insertion. It becomes slightly thicker again as it passes over the pars plana towards the cornea. In myopic and some normal eyes, the sclera is observably thinned and dark radial lines of black uvea show through the strips of thin sclera. There are bands of thin sclera situated between the annulus of muscle insertion and the equator. Scleral buckling procedures involve the insertion of intrascleral sutures, placement of which is much more difficult when the sclera is thin: superficial sutures tending to cut themselves out and deep ones to perforate the eye.

The surface of the sclera is criss-crossed by a delicate network of episcleral and scleral blood vessels. The anterior ciliary vessels enter the eye near the insertion of the rectus muscles. The exit of vortex veins through the sclera is by an oblique path and the overlying sclera often has a purple colour to warn of the presence of these delicate vessels. Injury to these vessels can give rise to choroidal haemorrhage and compromise intraocular circulation. The sclera is perforated posteriorly by the long ciliary nerves and the short ciliary arteries and nerves.

The sclera has little structural rigidity: the spherical shape of the eye is maintained partly by the intraocular pressure. While the sclera is malleable, it does not stretch or compress easily, thus a small rise in intraocular volume results in a marked rise in intraocular pressure. A temporary rise of intraocular pressure of 70 mmHg may occur with simple scleral indentation during indirect ophthalmoscopy or indentation with cryotherapy. These rises are temporary and usually unimportant, but the more sustained rise of intraocular pressure incurred when an explant is sutured on to an eye is more serious as it may stop intraocular perfusion altogether.

Anatomical Landmarks

External Landmarks (Fig. 1.3)

- Pars plana
- Ora serrata
- Vortex veins

The pars plana is the usual site for sclerotomies for vitrectomy and for intravitreal injection. The external landmark extends from 1.5 mm behind the limbus and extends posteriorly for up to 6 mm. A sclerotomy is usually made 3.5–4 mm behind the limbus.

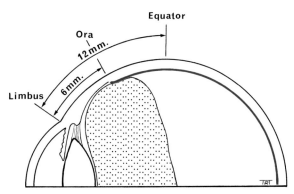

Fig. 1 3. Important surgical landmarks.

The ora serrata is marked by the ring of insertion of the rectus muscles and thus this muscle ring serves as a useful surface landmark for retinal dialysis. The location of the equator externally is approximately 14 mm behind the limbus.

The location of the vortex veins is variable and they exit the eye posterior to the equator. The vortex veins are found in greatest number on the nasal side, the upper half being favoured more than the lower. The upper temporal quadrant, which is the commonest quadrant for the surgeon to be operating upon, has only one vortex vein. Externally this is closely related to the tendon of the superior oblique muscle. The establishment of the site of the vortex veins (usually determined at the time of surgery because retinal detachment obscures them on pre-operative fundal examination) is important. If they are situated near retinal breaks they may be damaged during buckling or cryotherapy, and they may also be damaged if sited near the position where subretinal fluid is to be drained. Damage to veins can cause choroidal haemorrhage during surgery – the most feared operative complication.

Internal Landmarks (Fig. 1.4)

- Long ciliary nerves
- Short ciliary nerves and arteries
- Vortex veins ampullae
- Optic disc

The long ciliary vessels, which always accompany the long ciliary nerves, are found in two bundles. They are remarkably constant in their position,

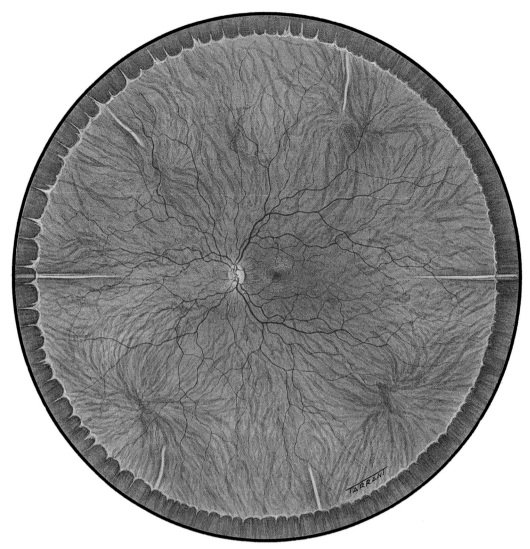

Fig. 14. The normal fundus.

being found in the horizontal meridian of each eye, dividing the retina into upper and lower parts, which helps surgical orientation. Each bundle emerges at the mid-point between the optic disc and the equator and is usually readily seen on a fundoscopy because of the increased pigmentation of the side of the bundles as they run forward. They should be avoided when the surgeon is working in the region of the horizontal rectus muscle. Although they may be damaged when buckling sutures are placed or

when subretinal fluid is being drained, damage to these structures seems rare in practice.

The short ciliary arteries are more irregular and variable in appearance than long ciliary arteries and are quite often not seen. They are usually situated around the vertical meridian. The short ciliary nerves are seen as whitish marks on the fundus and are often unaccompanied by the arteries which are more difficult to see. These vessels are of little significance to the surgeon.

The vortex veins vary considerably in number and are readily seen in the lightly pigmented subject. The ampullae mark the equator of the eye. Retinal blood vessels serve as useful landmarks for the localisation of retinal breaks; a simple sketch can serve to localise retinal breaks, which can be difficult to find per-operatively. The optic disc in a normal eye is about 1.5 mm in diameter and the size of the optic disc is often used as a convenient way of describing the size of a choroidal or retinal lesion. The view through a standard +20-dioptre indirect lens is approximately 12 mm in diameter.

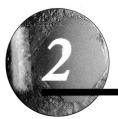

2 Examination of the Eye with Retinal Disease

The clinical examination of the eye with vitreo-retinal disease should follow a sequence of external examination, measurement of visual acuity, testing pupil reactions, slit-lamp examination of the anterior segment followed by indirect ophthalmoscopy with scleral indentation, and lastly with non-contact and occasionally contact lens biomicroscopy. The features of retinal detachment need to be recorded on retinal charts. These basic steps may be succeeded in some cases by special investigations including imaging the eye with ultrasonography, radiography, CT and MR scanning and fluorescein angiography. The examination sequence may need to be modified when examining special groups of patients such as children and mentally or physically disabled patients.

External Examination

A general ocular examination of both eyes is made with the object of excluding coexisting ocular disease before attention is turned specifically to the intraocular contents. Some eye conditions, such as ocular motility disorders, ptosis, proptosis and enophthalmos, may be better detected by external examination rather than with slit-lamp or indirect ophthalmoscopy. Similarly, extruding explants are usually deep in the fornices and patients may need to turn their eyes to extreme gaze in order to reveal the breach in the overlying conjunctiva. Sentinel vessels associated with a choroidal melanoma can be missed if the eye is observed through the relatively high magnification of the slit-lamp.

Measurement of Visual Acuity

A patient with an acute retinal detachment not involving the macula in an otherwise normal eye is expected to see 6/6 corrected. Patients with recent detachment of the macula can often still see as well as 6/18 provided the detachment is shallow. Patients may have poor central vision from other causes even when the retinal detachment does not involve the macula. Initial visual acuity is important in audit and outcome measurement; it is also of medicolegal importance and should be done on each occasion that the patient attends. No perception of light is not always a complete contraindication to surgery as sometimes absence of light perception is reversible (e.g. following trauma).

Ideally, the surgeon should measure the patient's vision personally, at least on the first visit. The fluency, accuracy and the confidence of the patient in reading the chart tells much about their disability. Symptoms such as distortion and blind spots, which are not easily quantified or measured, may be volunteered. Fresh intragel haemorrhage may not reduce the visual acuity and given time and with searching movement, many patients can catch a glimpse of the chart by looking though a relatively clear vista in the vitreous gel. A patient may record good visual acuity in the presence of gel opacities such as haemorrhage or hyalosis when the surgeon can only obtain a poor view of the retina. In contrast, retro-hyaloid haemorrhage can often obscure vision even when the bleed has been slight. Similarly, following a vitrectomy, an eye is essentially a fluid-filled compartment and any blood becomes diffuse and reduces vision markedly.

Optometrists, general medical practitioners, and hospital eye services commonly employ the Snellen chart for measuring visual acuity. Patients with vitreo-retinal disease, however, often have poor central vision and a low visual acuity. On the Snellen chart there are fewer letters at the lower visual acuities and this makes measurements unreliable. There is also a huge gap between the level of 6/60 and level of counting fingers. It is recommended that patients with poorer visual acuity be tested at a reduced distance of say 1 metre. A visual acuity recorded as 1/60 is more probably more reliable than one noted as Hand Movements. Similarly a vision of 1/18 is more informative than <6/60.

Increasingly in teaching hospital eye units, the EDTRS chart is being adopted. The chart is designed with equal number letters in each line and a logarithmic progression from one line to the next. It is more reliable for measuring low vision and more amenable to statistical analysis. It should be used if one wishes to measure subtle change in visual acuity from one occasion to another. Some types of vitreo-retinal surgery only produce marginal improvement in visual acuity, e.g. submacular surgery. The benefits might only be measurable using the EDTRS chart with a reduced working distance. The use of this chart pre- and post-operatively adds weight to scientific clinical studies (Fig. 2.1).

The Pupils

Of the many pupillary abnormalities, the vitreo-retinal surgeon is most interested in a defect in the integrity of the afferent pathway. The Swinging Torch Test is the most informative. Relative

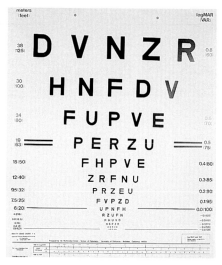

Fig. 2.1. The EDTRS chart.

Afferent Pupil Defects (RAPD) are best elicited using a relatively strong light, e.g. that provided by the indirect ophthalmoscope is convenient. Patients are examined in a darkened room and asked to fix in the distance. Although this is a test for the consensual light reflex, one only needs to observe the eye that is illuminated by the light (Fig. 2.2).

A positive RAPD is given by the paradoxical reaction of a pupil dilating when light is shone through it. A positive reaction is also given by the constriction of pupil of the contralateral unaffected eye. This latter sign is less reliable because often there is a momentary dilatation of the pupil as the torch is swung from one eye to the other. The normal reaction of the pupil to the Swinging Torch Test is a slight constriction. Nonetheless, if the pupil of the affected side is unavailable for examination because of iris damage, efferent defect or mydriasis, and the reaction of the fellow eye is that of marked constriction, then an RAPD should be strongly suspected.

The RAPD test is sensitive for optic nerve disease but is not particularly so for retinal detachment. Essentially it compares one eye with another and the pupil response to light is a mass reaction from the whole retina. For example, it may not reliably detect a peripheral retinal detachment if the macula is not detached although as much as half the retina may be elevated. Similarly, a patient with atrophic macular degeneration and a vision of 6/60 in one eye and 6/6

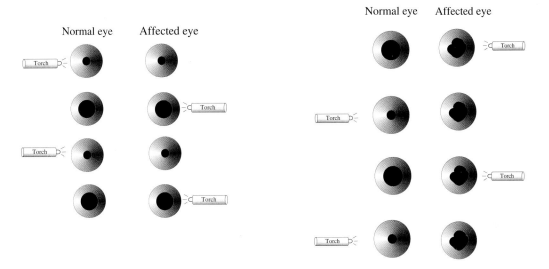

Fig. 2.2. Pupil reactions.

in the fellow eye may not exhibit an RAPD. This might be due to the fact that both maculae are affected by age-related changes although the actual visual acuity is very different. It is also important to appreciate that the presence of media opacity such as cataract formation or vitreous haemorrhage does not normally give rise to a RAPD when a bright light source is used. If an RAPD is present, it is vital to carry out ultrasound to elucidate the cause for the decreased sensory input on the affected side.

However, the availability of special investigations such as ultrasonography, electrodiagnostic tests and magnetic resonance scans does not diminish the importance of the clinical test of pupil reactions. A reliable positive RAPD sign carries considerable weight in establishing a diagnosis and in deciding upon treatments.

Slit-Lamp Examination

Using the slit-lamp, the examination of the cornea, anterior chamber, lens, iris, diaphragm, retro-lental space and the anterior vitreous is made.

Examination of the anterior third of the vitreous for its cellular content, state of degeneration and whether or not vitreous detachment is present, is enhanced by setting the gel in motion by asking the patient to look up and down. The vitreous may be optically empty in Stickler Syndrome cases.

Details of other anterior segment findings are given in Chap. 4.

Indirect Ophthalmoscopy and Scleral Depression

Examination of the retina should be conducted in a darkened room using indirect ophthalmoscopy and scleral indentation, and sufficient time should be given for the examination to be performed adequately. The posterior two thirds of the vitreous cavity and the vitreo-retinal interfaces are examined with contact and non-contact lenses. Indirect ophthalmoscopy is the most important clinical skill upon which a vitreo-retinal surgeon relies for the assessment and treatment of retinal detachment. Proficiency with its use requires a basic understanding of the optics. Direct and indirect ophthalmoscopy and biomicroscopy using say a +90 dioptre lens all make use of Gullstrand optics. In essence, the illumination beam and the line of sight must be separated by an angle; otherwise, specular reflection would prevent viewing. The smaller the angle of separation between the illumination and line of sight, the more glare will be reflected back from the examination lens, the cornea and the crystalline lens. For the direct ophthalmoscope, the angle of separation is determined by the slight tilt of the mirror reflecting light into the pupil. This angle is relatively small. The fundus is seen even when the pupil is relatively small. Viewing is monocular and there is no depth perception. The image is erect, virtual and relatively large and the field is relatively small. For the indirect ophthalmoscope, a triangle is formed at the pupil by the illuminating beam and two lines of sight one for each eye of the observer. This triangle is relatively large and the pupil needs to be correspondingly dilated to admit this triangle. A smaller pupil means that either the illuminating beam is admitted and there is no view, or the lines of sight are admitted and the field is dark. The use of the hand held lens forms a real, inverted image in free space a few inches from the observer. The +3.00 eye pieces incorporated in ophthalmoscope permit comfortable viewing. (Fig. 2.3 a,b)

Viewing Peripheral Retina: Basic Principles

With a widely dilated pupil, viewing of the posterior pole is not a problem. When the eye being examined is looking to one side, as when the peripheral retina is examined, the pupil changes from a round to an oval aperture. It becomes difficult to view the retina binocularly but it is possible to use the ophthalmoscope as a monocular instrument. To do this, the observer aligns the illuminating light beam and the line of sight of one eye along the long axis of

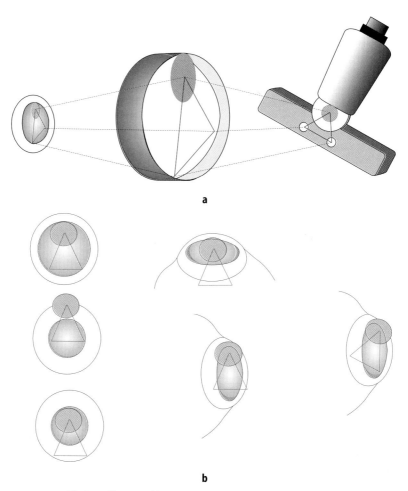

a

b

Fig. 2.3. a The optics of the indirect ophthalmoscope; **b** small pupil viewing.

the patient's pupil. It is essential for the observer to be correctly positioned to facilitate the examination. For example, to see the superior periphery of the right eye, the examiner should be standing on the patients right side and tilt his head to align the one limb of the triangle to fit into the oval projection of the pupil (Fig. 2.3b). The examiner moves around the patient who needs to be lying down. This basic technique combined with scleral indentation should allow complete examination of the pre-equatorial retina up to and including the ora serrata (Fig. 2.4).

Optics of Viewing through Small Pupils

There are modifications to the modern indirect ophthalmoscope that have made viewing the periphery easier. Some ophthalmoscopes are fitted with an adjustment for bringing together the two lines of sight. This reduces the base of the triangle enabling binocular viewing of the peripheral retina. This is at the expense of stereopsis as the two eyes of the observers are effectively brought closer together by the use of prisms. This adjustment should however, not be confused with the adjustment for inter-pupillary distance. Other ophthalmoscopes move the illuminating light beam closer to the two eye-

pieces for small pupil viewing. This reduces the height of the triangle. The illuminating light beam usually needs to be narrower otherwise specular reflection causes glare. Thus, a narrower illuminating beam for peripheral viewing or for small pupils is chosen.

The correct use of the hand lens can also help viewing of the peripheral retina. These are powerful converging lenses and as such have a prismatic effect. The lenses are usually placed centrally over the pupil for viewing the posterior retina. When examining the pre-equatorial retina, the lens is placed eccentrically to make use of the prismatic effect. The rule is to move the lens towards the direction of gaze. If the patient's eye is looking upward as when the superior retina is examined, then displacing the hand-held lens upwards slightly will bring into view more of the peripheral retina. The more powerful the hand-held lens, the greater is this prismatic effect. Using the more powerful hand-held lenses (the +28 D or the +30 D instead of the usual +20 D lens) will converge the beam and minify the triangle when projected into the pupil, thereby allowing the retina to be viewed through smaller pupils.

Magnification and Image Size

The image of the retina through more powerful lenses is smaller. By adjusting the observing distance, magnification of smaller image can be obtained through a given hand-held lens. The rule is to move the observer's head closer and the hand-held lens closer to the patient's eye to obtain a larger image. By moving closer to the patient, the real and inverted image in space is closer to the ophthalmoscope and greater magnification is achieved by accommodation of the examiner's own eyes.

Choice of Hand-held Lenses

A +20 dioptre lens gives the best compromise in terms of the size of image obtained, stereopsis and the ability to see through a reasonably dilated pupil without being monocular. The +28 dioptre hand-held lens is better for smaller pupils especially for viewing the periphery and is particularly useful in

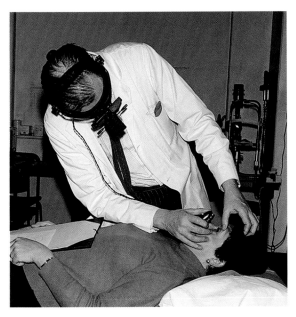

Fig. 2.4. Indirect ophthalmoscopy. Note the examiner's head tilt

gas-filled eyes and for the examination of small children.

Scleral Indentation

There are two main purposes for this examination:

- It allows viewing of peripheral retina.
- It introduces a dynamic aspect to the examination to facilitate break detection and pre-surgical planning.

Examination of the fundus should start at the periphery allowing time for the patients to become adjusted to the relatively bright light. This illumination should be turned down to view the macula. Be kind with the light, which can seem unbearable to a patient with a fully dilated pupil and positively searing to another with an inflamed eye. No fundal view is possible when the patient's eye is tightly shut! Indirect ophthalmoscopy should be performed initially without scleral indentation. It is only when the patient has become adjusted to the bright light and is at ease that scleral depression should be used.

Techniques of Scleral Indentation

When a patient is asked to look up or down, the lid sulcus becomes deep and virtually obliterated and it is difficult and often painful to insinuate the indentator into this sulcus. With the eye in the primary position, more of the equator of the eye is exposed and it is relatively easy to indent patients even those with deep-set eyes. The trick is not to ask the patient to look in extreme gaze, but for the examiner to tilt his head to achieve peripheral viewing. Gentle indentation is all that is necessary to bring the equatorial retina into view. To see the ora serrata, the patient is asked to look further up down or sideways. This automatically brings the anterior retina into view without moving the scleral depressor. The view of the 3 and 9 o'clock positions opposite the medial or lateral canthus are exposed and indentation through the lid is impossible. This can usually be circumvented by asking the patient to look slightly up or down. The experienced ophthalmoscopist appreciates that the more gentle is the indentation, the more is seen of the periphery.

Break Detection and Assessment

Scleral indentation helps with the detection of retinal breaks. (Fig. 2.5) This applies particularly to the case of retinal tears with overlying opercula. In highly detached retina, the operculum can obscure the view of a small U-shaped tear. It is only by scleral indentation and distorting the overlying retina that the 'lid' is displaced to reveal the opening. Small atrophic holes can easily be missed but for scleral indentation. By mounting these holes on the indent, the presence of the hole will be demonstrated as a small gap in the retina when it is seen in profile. Conversely, a retinal dialysis can be closed easily by the scleral depression and escape detection. A gap in the anterior insertion of the retina is only revealed by observing the down-slope on either side of the indent.

The scleral depressor, the tip of which is approximately 5 mm in width enables an estimate to be made of the size of the buckle required to close the retinal break. The ability to approximate pigment epithelium to neuro-epithelium helps to decide whether a non-drainage operation can be performed.

Biomicroscopy Using Non-Contact and Three-Mirror Contact Lenses

Non-contact hand-held lenses have several advantages:

- Allow binocular viewing of the retina at high magnification.
- Allow a view of the retina through small pupils.
- Acceptable to patient.

The disadvantages include:

- The illuminated field of view through small pupils is small and is inefficient for a complete survey of the retina.
- The more powerful lenses (e.g. +90 D) have poor axial magnification and it can be difficult to detect subtle elevation of the retina (e.g. clinically significant oedema).

Like the indirect ophthalmoscope, biomicroscopy using the hand-held lenses relies on Gullstrand

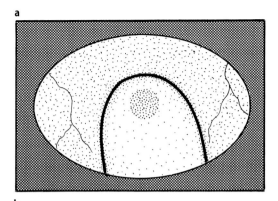

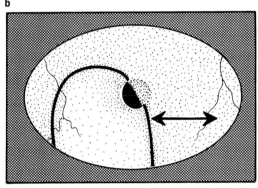

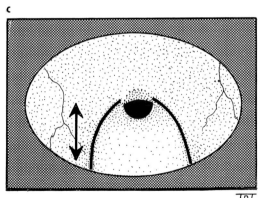

Fig. 2.5a–c. Scleral depression. Radial and circumferential movement of the depressor aids break detection.

optics. Although it is possible to obtain a view of the retina through a small pupil, the illuminated area needs to be small to avoid specular reflection. For a thorough survey of the whole retina, mydriasis is mandatory.

The hand-held lenses are useful tools for examination of the posterior pole. The +90 dioptre lens and the +78 provide a wide field of view. They are useful for the detection of shallow retinal detachments, macular holes, perivascular or peripapillary breaks in the high myope. The +60 lenses give slightly better axial magnification and are used for detecting subtle elevation of the retina.

Hand-held lenses may be useful in photocoagulation of patients who are intolerant of contact lenses.

Three-mirror contact lens examination has the following advantages but is used much less today:

- Magnification allows small break detection.
- Magnification allows break detection when the choroidal reflex has been diminished by previous surgery
- Axial magnification is useful for detecting shallowly elevated macular lesions

The difficulties in three-mirror examinations are:

- The contact lens is not particularly well tolerated in recently operated eyes.
- Severe squeezing interferes with the examination.

The three-mirror examination provides a view of the periphery at a higher magnification than that afforded by any of the hand held lenses. It is useful for the detection of small breaks, and especially suitable for cases in which the choroidal reflex has been whitened by previous retinopexy.

The central area through a Goldmann three-mirror lens can also be helpful in assessing macular disease, e.g. macular holes and cystoid macular oedema. Although the same view can be obtained using +90 lens, the Goldmann lens gives greater axial magnification. Subtle elevation of the retina associated with the cuff of subretinal fluid around a stage III macular hole or foveolar detachment in stage I disease can be detected. The most obtuse of the three mirrors also provides view of the anterior chamber angle and can provide a useful assessment of patients with coincidental glaucoma.

Three-mirror examination should not be performed within hours of surgery as it may make the cornea somewhat hazier and interfere with surgery.

Retinal Charts

A retinal drawing is made of the eye with retinal detachment prior to surgery. By thus identifying breaks and other landmarks, the time spent by the surgeon in becoming completely familiar with the retina to be operated upon will result in much saving of time during the operation itself. Making a chart obviates against the temptation for a cursory fundal examination prior to surgery. Charts are also useful

- As a learning exercise to the ophthalmologist in training as it ensures a commitment of physical signs to a formal record.
- As a research record
- As a medico-legal record.

The assessment of the findings of indirect ophthalmoscopy is often confusing to the beginner, the view of the retina being vertically inverted and laterally reversed by the indirect ophthalmoscope. This preoperative difficulty is overcome by placing the retinal chart on the patient in the upside down position during the examination. Thus, when the patient looks down with the surgeon standing above, details of the inferior retina will be indicated on the part of chart nearest the surgeon (and this will correspond to inferior retina in the transposed retinal chart). As the surgeon moves progressively around the eye, further details will be added sequentially to the chart.

When the retinal detachment has been accurately charted, it should be possible to form a clear-cut idea of what needs to be done at surgery. If there is a period of bed-rest before operation, it will be necessary to re-examine the retina before surgery. If subretinal fluid has been redistributed by bed-rest, the appearance of the retinal detachment may have changed dramatically, and the surgeon will need to be familiarised with the new conditions prior to operation.

Direct Ophthalmoscopy

Direct ophthalmoscopy is of little use in examining the detached retina but on occasions may be of help in patients with small pupils. Its role has largely been replaced by slit-lamp biomicroscopy using hand-held lenses.

Visual Fields

Visual fields have little part to play in the diagnosis of retinal detachment or other vitreo-retinal surgical disorders. The peripheral field will only start to become affected when retinal detachment has extended posterior to the equator. Visual fields are sometimes used to document the extent of peripheral visual loss associated with retinoschisis.

Transillumination

Transillumination is of value in distinguishing between a rhegmatogenous and a solid non-rhegmatogenous retinal detachment. A cold light source should be used and the guarded light pipe should be applied directly on the anaesthetised cornea to give a good result. The lids should be well retracted to see the posterior limit of any solid lesion and the patient should be asked to look in extreme gaze. Transillumination gives supportive evidence of a solid lesion to imaging by ultrasonography.

Examining Children

In rare cases when retinal detachment occurs in very young children, the examination poses particular problems. The child may be uncooperative and is usually apprehensive. This apprehension may be partially relieved by the presence of a calm parent. In these conditions, the examination must not be allowed to take too long and the subject's confidence in the examiner must be built up slowly. Similarly, mentally disabled patients are unable to give their full co-operation. With patience, it may be possible to examine the retina in detail. Only the very gentlest scleral depression should be practised, indeed, often it is not possible to do so at all. In many cases, it is only possible to make a general examination of the fundus and a detailed examination has to be deferred until the patient is anaesthetised. Indirect ophthalmoscopic examination can be made with scleral depression and a fundal chart completed in the operating room.

Special Investigations

After a basic clinical examination, special investigations may be necessary. There are limited and specific indications for radiography but where fundal view is seriously impaired ultrasonography is mandatory.

The need to carry out assessment of vitreo-retinal surgical conditions complicated by opaque media is a frequent occurrence. Ultrasonography should be within the competence of every retinal surgeon.

Ultrasonography

The skills of performing the ultrasound examination and interpretation of the findings can be acquired by the vitreo-retinal surgeon through practice. Scanners should therefore be easily available where patients are examined. Conditions identified by ultrasonography need to be confirmed by the findings at surgery and this feedback is essential in building up confidence in diagnosis.

The Basic Principles of Ultrasonography

Ultrasonography uses pezo-electric crystals to generate a beam of ultrasound wave (interrogating beam) directed into the eye and orbit. A transducer is used to 'listen' to the echoes of sound waves reflected back by the different structure within the globe (reflected beam). The strength of the echoes reflected back from an interface between two structures depends on the impedance, which in turn depends on the difference in the velocity of the ultrasound travelling from one medium into another. The healthy vitreous gel is relatively homogenous and produces little echo. The strength of the reflected ultrasound wave depends also on the angle of incidence and reflection. If an ultrasound beam is incident almost at right angles to an interface, more of the beam will be reflected back to the transducer to produce an echo. Thus, dynamic studies are necessary to detect mobile structures in order to present surfaces perpendicular to the interrogating ultrasound beam. With eye movement, structures with low impedance such as the posterior vitreous face can be seen.

Equipment Setting

For vitreo-retinal assessment B-mode ultrasonography is commonly used. Modern B mode ultrasound scan either make use of an array of transducers or motorised transducers to give an oscillatory or rotatory sweep and provide good lateral resolution. For vitreo-retinal work a 10-MHz weakly focused probe gives the best images. Most scanners have controls to modulate and enhance the echoes from deeper structure. The profile of this enhancement is given by the gain curve, which can be adjusted to give better resolution of the structures within the vitreous cavity.

Performing the Scan

It is important to adopt a standard approach and perform the scan in a set sequence.

The ultrasound probe is clearly annotated to indicate the direction of scanning and its orientation with respect to the display on the monitor. The patient being can be examined seated or supine. Sufficient coupling gel should be used to provide good contact. The patient should be asked to look down with eyes opened and the probe should be applied to the upper lid. The upper part of the fundus is best examined through the lower lid and with the eye looking up. Horizontal scans are usually taken to build up a three-dimensional image in the clinician's mind. Additional vertical and oblique scans may give extra information. Although modern scanners have good lateral resolution, the best image is acquired with the centre of the beam. If the area of interest is the upper nasal quadrant, the patient should be asked to look up and nasally. The largest cross section of the globe should be obtained. With dynamic B mode, cross sections including the optic nerve will confirm the eye movement and the mobility of other structures can be assessed relative to the eye movements.

The way a structure moves also give valuable information as to its identity. Vitreous gel with a completed vitreous detachment moves in a characteristic undulating pattern. The movement of the posterior vitreous face lags behind movement of the eye wall and typically continues to move when the eye stops. The movement of retro-hyaloid blood can best be described as Brownian. Fine 'speckles' of echoes from blood cells seem to move in random directions wafted along by intraocular currents. The vitreous gel can sometimes be ultrasonically silent and the detached vitreous gel can be highlighted as 'negative' image by retro-hyaloid blood; the vitreous gel occupies the vitreous cavity where there are no echoes. The presence of retro-hyaloid blood may therefore be useful when assessing the extent of posterior vitreous detachment in cases of proliferative diabetic retinopathy.

Interpretation of Ultrasound Findings

When interpreting the ultrasound images, consider the following:

1. Other findings on clinical examination.
2. Familiarise the images obtained by standard setting .
3. Use image processing to get more information.
4. Change the settings where appropriate.
5. Beware of artefacts, e.g. intraocular lenses, foreign bodies and internal tamponade agents.

The interpretation of the findings on ultrasonography needs to take into account the history and physical signs elicited on clinical examination. The mode of visual loss, the level of vision, gross examination of visual field and pupil reaction all contribute to establish the diagnosis. For example, a common diagnostic difficulty with ultrasonography is the distinction between vitreous and retinal detachment. In cases of longstanding vitreous

haemorrhage, the posterior vitreous face could give rise to high echoes, which might be confused with a total retinal detachment. If there was a marked afferent pupil defect then the weight of evidence would point to a retinal detachment.

Many ultrasound scanners permit processing of the ultrasound image after it has been acquired. Weak signals can be boosted and may highlight features hidden by surrounding high echoes. For example, reducing the power of the interrogating ultrasound beam can sometimes reveal pathological calcification or foreign bodies. The permutations of setting provide more information from a given captured image. The clinician should however get used to the appearance of normal and pathological structures with a standardised setting. The interpretations of the scans need to be validated by feedback obtained from operative findings before experimenting with altering the appearances of the scanned images. By changing the setting from case to case, it can be confusing to interpret the scans. Vitreous face can be adjusted to appear as retina and vice versa. Most scanners allowed a set of standardised settings to be saved such that the same settings will be available on starting the machine each time.

Image Artefacts: Pattern Recognition

The following conditions produce clearly identifiable patterns:

- Fresh retinal detachment
- Posterior vitreous detachment
- Longstanding retinal detachments
- Choroidal detachments
- Diabetic vitreous haemorrhage
- Vitreous incarceration
- Uveitis, retro-hyaloid blood, emulsified silicone oil droplets, asteroid hyalosis
- Trauma and intraocular foreign bodies
- Solid detachments
- Phthisis bulbi

Much of the interpretation of ultrasound images of the eye is about pattern recognition.

PVD and Retinal Detachment

A freshly detached vitreous gel has a free undulating movement and the posterior vitreous face is recognised by a weakly echogenic interface mapping out a sinusoidal wave like motion (Fig. 2.6a). A retinal detachment has a stronger echo and is recognised by its insertion at the disc and the ora serrata. A long-standing retinal detachment (Fig. 2.6b) assumes a triangular configuration with reduced mobility. In advanced cases, the leaves of the retina are seen to be apposed in front of the optic nerve head. The freshly detached retina with a bullous configuration has a similar pattern to the detached vitreous gel but the gel itself is often visible anterior to it. Sometimes a cross section of the vitreous cavity can slice across two or more folds of highly detached retina and give rise to a confusing picture with multiple echo interfaces on the scans.

Choroidal Detachment (Fig. 2.6c)

Choroidal detachments usually extend into the pars plana and characteristically give rise to a more vertical angle than retinal detachment. The detached choroid moves with eye movement and a give rise to a juddering rather than the undulating motion more typical of the vitreous or retina. Very rarely, one can also image the neuro-vascular bundle of the long ciliary nerves and vessels.

Proliferative Diabetic Retinopathy (Fig. 2.6d)

In eyes with proliferative diabetic retinopathy, especially those with fundal view obscured by vitreous haemorrhage, B-mode scan is helpful in determining the extent of posterior vitreous detachment and assessing the complexity of tractional retinal detachment. Such information will be useful for surgical planning. In an eye with a first time vitreous haemorrhage, the diabetic hyaloid is almost invariably attached at the disc; this helps to differentiate it from other causes of haemorrhage such as posterior vitreous detachment and retinal tears.

Trauma and Intraocular Foreign Bodies

In severe posterior segment injury, ultrasound investigation can reveal anatomical disruption including vitreous incarceration, the presence of choroidal detachment, suprachoroidal blood and the position and integrity of the crystalline lens. By its very nature, ultrasonography is not efficient in detecting foreign bodies. Even with serial sections, it is difficult to be sure that every aspect of the eye has been interrogated. Because of their geometric shape, a foreign body can scatter ultrasound beam and thereby escape detection. Where a foreign body is radio-opaque a CT scan would be the investigation of choice.

Uveitis, Retro-hyaloid Blood, Silicone Oil Droplets and Asteroid Hyaloids

High speckled echoes are produced in posterior uveitis by cellular infiltration of the vitreous cavity (Fig. 2.6e). Similarly, asteroid hyalosis produces strong speckled echoes and highlights the movement of detached vitreous gel. Another example of high speckled echoes is provided for by emulsified droplets. These droplets are suspended in a fluid-filled cavity and adopt the Brownian movements, in all directions, not dissimilar to those produced by retro-hyaloid blood.

Solid Detachments

Ultrasound examination is also useful in the differential diagnosis of solid detachment. The clinical differential diagnosis is between choroidal haemangioma, metastatic deposits, malignant choroidal melanoma and a disciform subretinal neovascularisation complex. This task can be made more difficult in the presence of an obscured media. For example, disciform membranes can bleed into the vitreous cavity obscuring fundal view. Ultrasound examination of these cases often reveals the presence of Bruch's membrane rupture. This is shown on the ultrasound scans as two echoes on either side of the lesion forming an acute angle with the retinal surface. A break through the basement membrane of the retina is also observed with choroidal melanoma. In these instances, the melanoma often has a collar stud appearance. A choroidal melanoma with an intact overlying Bruch's membrane usually has a hemispherical shape and the lesion can be either ultrasonically solid or empty. Choroidal excavation is sometimes detected. Metastatic deposits are usually located in the posterior pole and generally have irregular shape and a low profile.

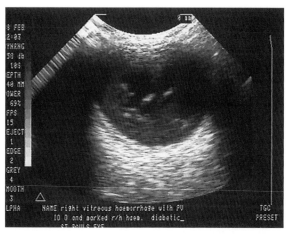
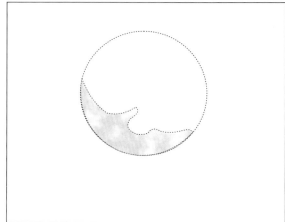

Part i

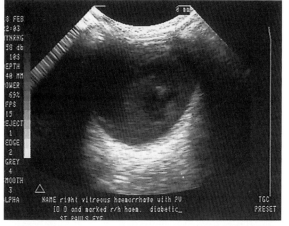
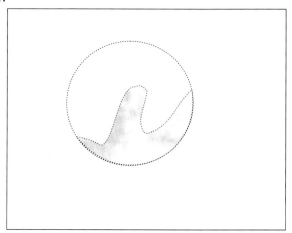

Part ii

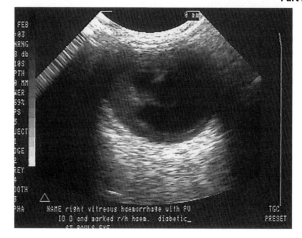
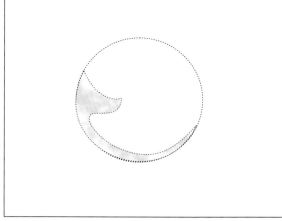

Part iii

Fig. 2.6. Various ultrasounds. **a** PVD highlighted by retro-hyaloid blood (parts i–iii this page, part iv opposite).

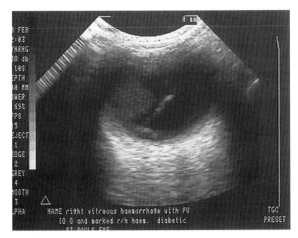
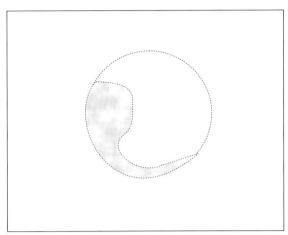

Fig. 2.6a. Part iv.

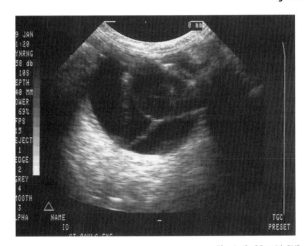
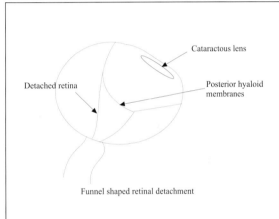

Fig. 2.6b. RD, with PVR triangular configuration.

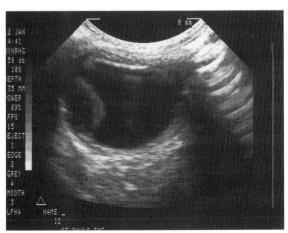
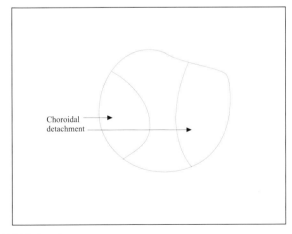

Fig. 2.6c. Choroidal detachment.

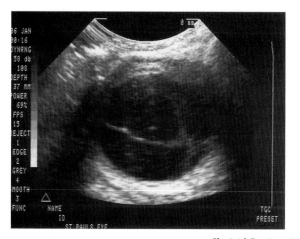 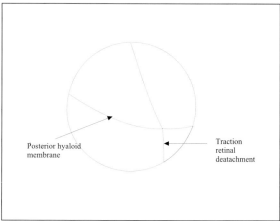

Fig. 2.6d. Traction retinal detachment in PDR.

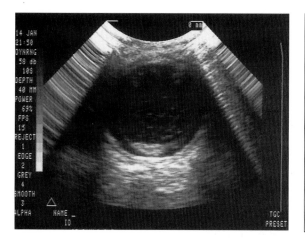 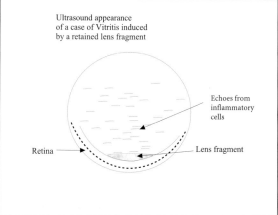

Fig. 2.6e. Uveitis from dropped lens fragments.

Simply because a lesion is ultrasonically empty does not mean that it is a cystic lesion and that it is not as it were a 'solid' detachment. The absence of echoes within the lesion simply indicates the tissue is ultrasonically homogenous. This is taken to indicate slow growth. Rapid tumour growth can be associated with areas of necrosis within the lesion as the tumour outgrows its blood supply. The tumour become ultrasonically heterogeneous and produces high echoes within the lesion.

Phthisis Bulbi

Grossly thickened eye walls presumably from congested choroid in small globes with retinal detachments indicate phthisis.

Image Artefacts

There are a number of image artefacts of which to be wary. Intraocular lenses present a large specular reflecting surface to an interrogating ultrasound beam. It can cause ringing echoes like a hall of mirrors with the ultrasound beam bouncing backwards and forwards between the lens surface and the transducer. The crystalline lens can also cause distortion of image. The velocity of ultrasound through the lens is faster than through vitreous and the interrogating beam is refracted as well as reflected (Baum's bumps). The surface of the retina appears as a saucer shaped elevation behind the crystalline lens. Irregular shaped foreign bodies scatter as well as absorb the ultrasound beam and can give rise to ultrasonic shadows. Some foreign bodies are identified by the shadow they cast rather than by the high echoes produced at the site where they are located. The presence of internal tamponade agents can cause difficulty in imaging the structures of the eye. Ultrasound energy is absorbed by gas and usually this 'blocks' the ultrasound beam from interrogating structures lying behind a bubble. The velocity through silicone oil is greatly reduced and the time lapse between sending an interrogating wave and receiving its echoes is increased. This gives an artificially lengthened image of the eye. B-mode ultrasonography of silicone-filled eyes is of very limited value.

> Do your own ultrasonography and learn to recognise the different patterns.

X-Ray and Computerised Tomography

When ocular penetration has occurred and an intraocular foreign body is suspected a full clinical examination including indirect ophthalmoscopy should be carried out through dilated pupils before

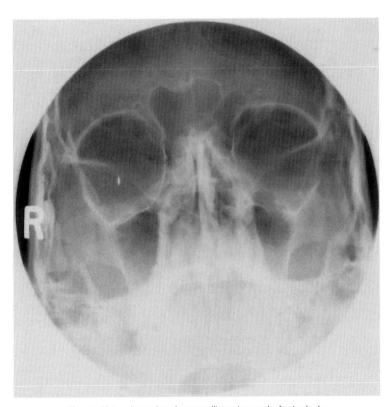

Fig. 2.7. Plain radiograph to show metallic eye intraocular foreign body.

considering special investigations. The fundal view is often obscured by media opacity such as cataract and vitreous haemorrhage. A plain radiograph (Fig. 2.7) will confirm the presence and number of radio-opaque foreign bodies including glass with a high lead content. CT imaging of the eye is the only effective method of determining whether a radio-opaque foreign body is in the vitreous cavity, impacted in the eye wall or outside the globe when a fundal view cannot be obtained. A precise know-ledge of the location of the foreign body is import-ant for the planning of surgery for its removal. (Fig. 2.8)

MRI

MRI is useful for the detection of non-metallic foreign bodies. (Fig. 2.9)

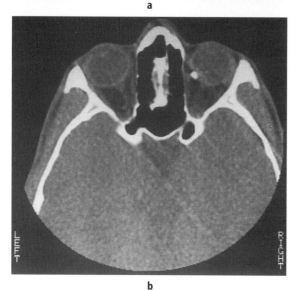

Fig. 2.8. CT scan to show: **a** intraocular foreign body; **b** extraocular foreign body.

Fluorescein Angiography

Fluorescein angiography is of little help in the diagnosis or assessment of rhegmatogenous retinal detachment but may be helpful in a variety of other conditions with which the vitreo-retinal surgeon may be involved. Exudative retinal detachment is an important differential diagnosis in some cases of retinal detachment and fluorescein angio-graphy may be help in detecting Harada's diseases, choroidal effusion syndrome and sympathetic ophthalmia.

Macular Pathology

Angiography may be useful in cases of macular pucker, not only to detect whether the pucker is primary or secondary (e.g. to branch vein occlu-sion), but also to detect leakage from vessels and pigment epithelial damage that may indicate a worse prognosis. It is essential to define the extent and activity of submacular neovascularisation in cases in which surgery is contemplated. It helps in the differential diagnosis of full thickness macular hole, a clinical appearance of which can be mimicked by cystoid macular oedema or holes in epimacular membranes.

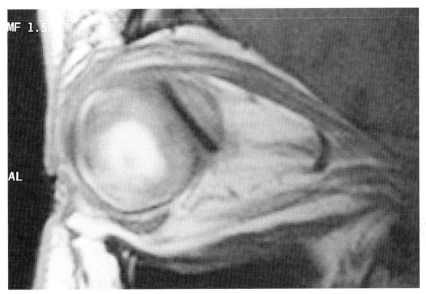

Fig. 2.9. NMR image of a non-metallic foreign body.

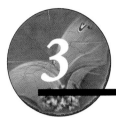

3

Rhegmatogenous Retinal Detachment (RRD): Pathogenesis and Clinical Features

Definition

Retinal detachment occurs when fluid accumulates between the photoreceptor and pigment epithelial cell layers of the retina; in rhegmatogenous retinal detachment (RRD) the fluid accumulates after a break has formed in the photoreceptor layer.

Incidence

RRD occurs in approximately 1 in 10 000 of the UK population per year.

Pathogenesis of RRD

In most cases the sequence of events resulting in RRD starts with vitreous degeneration which in turn causes vitreous collapse resulting in posterior vitreous detachment (PVD). PVD may produce traction on the underlying retina causing break formation or activation of an existing break. Fluid from the vitreous compartment enters the subretinal space via the

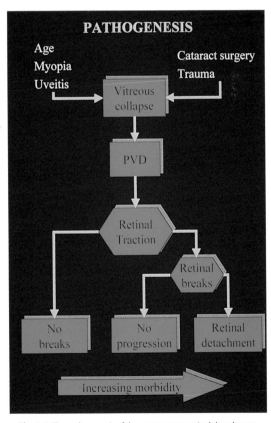

Fig. 3.1. The pathogenesis of rhegmatogenous retinal detachment.

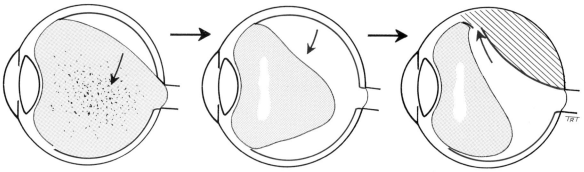

Fig. 3.2. The sequence of posterior vitreous detachment, retinal break formation and retinal detachment.

retinal break producing retinal detachment. The three main components of the pathogenesis of RRD (Fig. 3.1), vitreous detachment, break formation and the accumulation of subretinal fluid (SRF; Fig. 3.2), will now be considered in more detail.

Vitreous Detachment

Simple

Vitreous detachment occurs as a consequence of vitreous degeneration and collapse. It may be considered as a normal ageing change of the gel as approximately two out of three people over the age of 40 can be expected to develop vitreous detachment. The normal interaction between hyaluronic acid and the collagen content of the vitreous gel breaks down. The collagen fibrils tend to condense and the gel itself becomes more fluid. Spaces form within it (lacunae) and the normal vitreous architecture is lost. Any event that alters the normal gel structure will promote vitreous detachment (e.g. age, myopia, trauma, uveitis). Although the link between vitreous detachment and retinal detachment is clear, the mechanism of production and progression of vitreous detachment is still poorly understood. Separation from the disc induces a circular opacity in the posterior hyaloid face (Weiss ring). The presence of this opacity is the only sure way to diagnose complete posterior vitreous detachment. Vitreous may herniate backwards through dehiscences in the posterior hyaloid. Saccadic and other eye movements causing continual rotational movement of the gel results in pulling forces upon points of attachment – dynamic vitreo-retinal traction. Occasionally, vitreous detachment is

incomplete and the vitreous remains firmly adherent to the posterior pole and the macular region. This partial gel detachment may result in tractional retinal elevation of the macular area (the vitreomacular tractional syndrome).

Complex

Complex PVD occurs when vitreous separation arises in the presence of retinal disease, which prevents complete gel separation from the retinal surface. Points of firm attachment of gel to retina occur, for example, at neovascular complexes (Fig. 3.3a), choroidoretinal inflammatory foci and retina affected by trauma either contusive or penetrating. Progressive contraction of gel increases traction on these areas which may result in tractional retinal detachment, tractional retinoschisis or RRD. Mixed retinal pictures can occur. The occurrence of both simple and complex posterior vitreous detachment demonstrates that the posterior vitreous cortex has a pivotal role to play in the pathogenesis of surgical vitreo-retinal disease.

Presentation of Simple PVD

PVD may be symptomatic or asymptomatic.

Symptoms

Flashes of light, or floaters, or both are the symptoms of PVD. It is unusual for flashes to be experienced alone but floaters alone are common. Flashes usually but not invaribaly precede floaters.

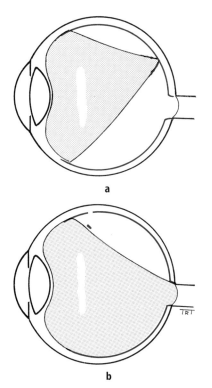

Fig. 3.3. a Complex vitreous detachment associated with retinal neovascularisation; **b** simple vitreous detachment and retinal break (hole) formation.

Flashes

White flashes of light attributed to vitreo-retinal traction are for an unknown reason usually experienced in the temporal field of vision. This may last a few seconds or may be experienced several times a day for a few days. As traction is relieved upon the retina, either due to spontaneous separation of the gel or if retinal detachment itself occurs, flashes usually disappear spontaneously. However, they sometimes persist for weeks or months.

Floaters

A detached posterior hyaloid becomes visible and results in a variety of shapes and sizes of opacity which move within the vitreous cavity, and are perceived as such by the patient.

In middle-aged or older patients flashes and floaters either alone or in combination suggest PVD

and urgent assessment is required to exclude retinal breaks. Flashes are the more important symptoms increasing the risk of break formation complicating PVD.

Reduction of Vision

Temporary reduction of vision may be caused by vitreous opacities subsequent to vitreous detachment or by vitreous haemorrhage if present. Although haemorrhage complicating PVD is usually insignificant with small punctate collections on the retinal surface, sometimes quite marked peripapillary haemorrhage or extensive bleeding into the gel occurs. In cases when vitreous haemorrhage occurs the incidence of retinal breaks is much higher than in cases not thus complicated.

Sequelae of PVD

Retinal breaks are produced in approximately 10–15% of cases of symptomatic PVD. PVD may also induce glial epiretinal-retinal membranes (e.g. macular pucker).

Symptoms of Complex PVD

Flashes of light are seldom experienced, but floaters caused by vitreous haemorrhage may occur.

> Sudden onset of flashes or floaters or both in patients over the age of approximately 40 years suggests PVD. Retinal breaks and impending RRD must be excluded.

Retinal Breaks (Fig. 3.4)

If a retinal break formed as a result of PVD (Fig. 3.3b) is to progress to RRD then usually it does so within a few days or weeks. Pigment granules can gain the vitreous cavity via the retinal break and may be detected in the retrolenticular space or later in gel (Schaffer's sign). Pigment is best seen when the gel is set in moton by looking up and down. In cases of PVD complicated by breaks and/or RRD pigment is always present. The production of a

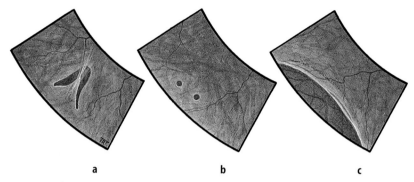

a   b   c

Fig. 3.4. Various types of retinal breaks: **a** retinal tear; **b** round holes; **c** retinal dialysis.

retinal break may result in bleeding from a retinal vessel producing haemorrhage into the vitreous cavity. This haemorrhage is variable in severity. Most usually it is not particularly so and is noticed by the patient as a shower of black spots. Less commonly, haemorrhage into the vitreous cavity may be severe causing profound reduction of vision and obscuration of retinal details. If a break has been present for months, then a ring of pigment may be found completely or incompletely surrounding it. Retinal breaks are described according to their shape, size or position.

Shape

By far the most commonly encountered breaks are either tears or holes. Tears are produced by vitreous failing to detach from the retina at a focal point of vitreous attachment, and the resulting traction produces a break with vitreous attached to the flap of the tear. These tears are commonly horseshoe-shaped, but may be irregular or slit-like. Retinal holes are produced either as a consequence of vitreous detachment when the detaching vitreous manages to avulse a piece of retina at a focal point of attachment, or may occur as consequence of retinal weakness, either at a point of degeneration (e.g. lattice degeneration), or in a patch of inflammation (e.g. CMV or acute retinal necrosis), or in apparently normal retina. Retinal tears favour the upper temporal quadrant in the myopic and non-myopic eye whereas holes are found more frequently in the lower temporal quadrant of the non-myopic eye. Thus the upper temporal quadrant is the one that the surgeon will be visiting most often in RRD surgery.

Size

This term may also be applied to certain types of breaks, e.g. giant breaks.

Position

This term is also used, e.g. macular holes.

Clinical Significance of Breaks

All breaks have to be sealed when they occur with RRD. The ease of detection and closure of these breaks will be an important factor in determining the complexity of the case, e.g. small breaks may be difficult to find, large ones difficult to close. For example, breaks at or anterior to the equator are more accessible to an external approach than breaks that are at the posterior pole.

Vitreous Haemorrhage

Vitreous haemorrhage may occur subsequent to posterior vitreous detachment alone, but more commonly complicates vitreous detachment associated with retinal break formation. Although it is wise to assume that any vitreous haemorrhage is caused by a retinal break until proved otherwise, other causes of vitreous haemorrhage have to be borne in mind. For example, caused by the vaso-proliferative retinopathies (diabetes, branch retinal vein occlusion, and HBSC disease) and other less common but usually obvious causes e.g., Terson's syndrome or trauma. The possibility of non-accidental injury should be considered in children.

Progression

The reason why some breaks proceed to RRD and others do not is poorly understood, and numerically the majority of retinal breaks do not lead to RRD. Tears are more likely to progress than holes and large breaks more likely to do so than small ones.

Formation and Spread of Subretinal Fluid (SRF)

Contour

As SRF accumulates the detaching retina assumes a convex configuration towards the vitreous, (and therefore towards the examiner) and also towards flat retina. This is in contrast to the concave contour both towards vitreous and flat retina when a tractional retinal detachment is present.

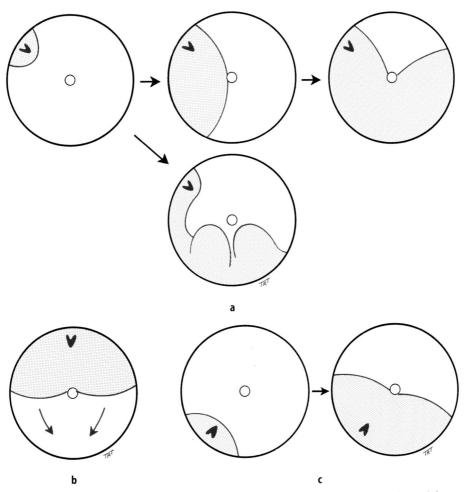

Fig. 3.5. Spread of SRF: **a** from a superior break resulting in either subtotal retinal detachment or in bullous inferior detachment; **b** from a superior midline break; **c** from an inferior break.

Direction of Spread of SRF

The direction of spread is predictable and SRF distribution conforms to the position of the primary retinal break in over 90% of cases. SRF accumulating around the retinal break spreads first to the ora serrata. Subsequent spread will be influenced by the position of the break in the retina, and by any obstructions in the natural pathway of the spread (e.g. areas of choroido retinal adhesion).

Superior Temporal and Superior Nasal Breaks (Fig. 3.5a)

Fluid descends on the same side as the break towards the disc, it then swings below the disc and with rapid progressive accumulation often resulting in inferior bullae will rise up again on the other side of the retina. However, It will, assume an upper level lower than that of the side from which it began.

Superior Midline Breaks

SRF from breaks situated near the midline (i.e. directly above the disc) will spread symmetrically down each side of the disc (Fig. 3.5b) The detachment becomes total. If the break is slightly to one side, the fluid front will be lower on the side co-incidental with the break. If the break is situated in a posterior position the SRF spread is somewhat more unreliable and the contour edges will be of less localising value. However, these breaks are easily seen.

Inferior Breaks

The detachment gradually rises to involve the macula, but rarely becomes total. The fluid will rise higher on the side of the retinal break and such detachments are never bullous (Fig. 3.5c).

SRF distribution is consistent with the site of the break.

Rate of Spread of SRF

Position of Break

SRF will accumulate quickly if the break is in the upper half of the retina, whereas with inferior breaks SRF accumulation is slower.

Size of Break

Retinal detachments with large breaks extend more rapidly than those with small breaks.

State and Position of the Vitreous

If the vitreous gel is of apparently normal consistency, e.g. in a young subject with a traumatic retinal detachment then the rate of progression of RRD will be slower than if the gel is degenerate (e.g. in myopia) or absent as in the vitrectomised eye.

SRF Formation

- Rapid: big breaks, superior position, degenerate or absent gel
- Slow: small breaks, inferior position, 'normal' gel

Shifting SRF

SRF which shifts its position markedly when the position of the head is altered indicates fluid which is denser in the subretinal than in the vitreal compartment. This sign is often a sign of non-rhegmatogenous detachment, but may also be seen in rhegmatogenous cases, particularly when retinal breaks are small and anterior, preventing free exchange of subretinal and vitreous fluid.

Natural History of RRD

Untreated RRD usually progresses until it is total. The retina becomes thin and atrophic and peri-retinal membranes infiltrate retina and vitreous. The normal undulating mobility of the retina is progressively lost. Less frequently RRD may become localised and static for many years, walled off by demarcation lines. Rarely spontaneous reattachment occurs. If the detachment is total, cataract usually develops after some months and eventually the eye tends to become phthisical; less commonly glaucoma develops. This downward chain of events is accelerated in cases that have been unsuccessfully treated.

Clinical Significance

Long-term detachment of the macula with disruption of the photoreceptor layer will result in poor restoration of central vision if reattachment is achieved.

Predisposing Factors

Retinal detachment has a strong bilateral tendency (about 20% of non-traumatic cases) and may occur in families. Factors which predispose to retinal detachment do so either by increasing the risk of posterior vitreous detachment or by weakening the retina directly. On some occasions both factors are present (e.g. lattice degeneration in a myopic eye).

Increased Risk of Simple PVD

- Myopia
- Cataract surgery
- Uveitis

Myopia

PVD and the peripheral retinal degenerative changes of lattice degeneration are more likely to be found in the large myopic eye. Retinal detachment occurs eight times more frequently in myopes than in the normal population, a risk that increases with the degree of myopia. High myopia with retinal detachment is more common in the male population than in the female, a tendency that is not found with the lower levels of myopia.

RRD risk factors
- Myopia
- Cataract surgery
- Uveitis
- Retinal weakness (degeneration or inflammation)
- Tractional retinal detachment (TRD)
- Trauma
- Family history

Cataract Surgery

There is a risk of retinal detachment following all forms of cataract surgery, although the mechanism of this relationship is not always clear. The risk of RRD following cataract extraction is now low due to preservation of the posterior capsule with either the extracapsular or the phacoemulsification techniques. Removal of the crystalline lens predisposes the eye to posterior vitreous detachment, a risk that is considerably increased if there has been a vitreous complication during the performance of the cataract operation or if YAG capsulotomy is subsequently performed. The risk is compounded if other predisposing factors such as myopia or lattice retinal degenerative changes are present. Retinal detachment may occur many years after the surgery of congenital cataract. This delay is related to the eventual occurrence of PVD.

Uveitis

Infiltration of white cells into the vitreous body causing degeneration and collapse increases the risk of PVD.

Causes of Retinal Breaks other than Simple PVD

1. Retinal degenerations (e.g. lattice or snail track degeneration) predispose an eye to break formation either prior to vitreous detachment when round holes may form or as in lattice degenera-

tion when tears are produced subsequent to PVD.

2. Inflammations. Inflammation of the retina (e.g. CMV retinitis) may weaken the retina and lead to break formation (in CMV these breaks are usually multiple, round and situated in the equatorial region of the retina). Vitreous detachment may or may not occur.

3. Tractional retinal detachment (TRD). Retinal breaks may be produced by sustained vitreo-retinal traction. The usual situation is a TRD complicating vaso-proliferative retinopathy (e.g. diabetes, HBSC disease, branch vein occlusion), the full thickness break may either remain static or add a rhegmatogenous component to the TRD.

4. Trauma. Trauma may cause retinal breaks, whether contusive or penetrating in nature. There is little evidence to support the notion that blows to other parts to the head may result in retinal detachment.

Contusive Injury

In contusive injury the globe is temporarily deformed at the moment of impact and although the walls of the globe are capable of movement the inelastic gel is not. (Fig. 3.6) The types of retinal breaks seen after contusion injuries reflect the various events that may happen at the vitreo-retinal interface following such an injury.

- Without vitreous detachment. The main effect occurs at the vitreous base, the walls of the eye moving away from the base result in the retinal break characteristic of contusive trauma, i.e. the

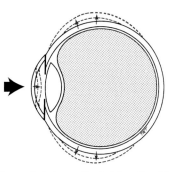

Fig. 3.6. Trauma. Contusion resulting in deformation of the globe.

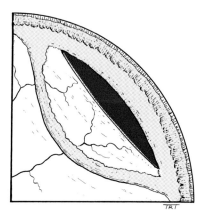

Fig. 3.7. Trauma. Avulsion of the vitreous base associated with retinal dialysis.

retinal dialysis (Fig. 3.7). The dialysis pathognomonic of ocular contusion is found in the upper nasal quadrant of the retina and is formed at the time of the injury. The role of trauma in the production of dialysis in the lower temporal quadrant is uncertain. In addition to dialyses, sudden movement of the gel in the region of the vitreous base may result in avulsion of the vitreous base and cause slit-like breaks in the pars plana. Other breaks that are sometimes seen without vitreous detachment are large round holes which form in areas previously affected by commotio retinae.

- Acute posterior vitreous detachment. Sudden gel movement from the posterior pole may produce macular breaks or large irregular paravascular tears.
- Delayed posterior vitreous detachment may result in equatorial breaks.

Perforating Injury

In scleral injuries (either self-sealing or open lacerations), posterior to the ora serrata retinal breaks without vitreous detachment are usually produced adjacent to the entry site (Fig. 3.8), or at the other side of the globe at a site of impaction or double perforation by a foreign body. More unusually breaks may be produced some weeks later due to delayed posterior vitreous detachment. Perforation of the globe by a needle being used for peri- or retro-bulbar anaesthesia may cause entry and exit site retinal breaks.

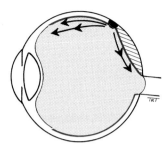

Fig. 3.8. Trauma. Posterior incarceration results in traction due to gel and retinal incarceration.

Methods of Presentation of RRD

Flashes of light and floaters are caused by vitreous detachment and these are succeeded by a field defect if RRD occurs subsequent to break formation. The timing and presence of all three symptoms is variable and only 50% of patients suffering from RRD have any of them.

The three 'Fs' of RRD
● Flashes
● Floaters
● Field defects

1. Flashes of light. Flashes of light due to vitreo-retinal traction are usually experienced in the temporal field of vision and do not localise the site of the retinal break.
2. Floaters. These are perceived as mobile opacities and usually appear after the onset of flashes if both are present. However, if vitreous haemorrhage (usually subsequent to break formation) has occurred, they may vary from a shower of black spots to extensive loss of vision. This haemorrhage is usually a singular event, but is sometimes repeated over months or years. Blood may be found in retro-hyaloid, or intravitreal compartments or both.
3. Field defect. A defect develops when the retinal detachment extends posterior to the equator and therefore RRD may be extensive before a field defect is noticed. An inferior nasal field defect indicates an RRD starting from the superior temporal quadrant and an inferior temporal defect indicates one from the superior nasal quadrant. Superior defects, detected much less readily than inferior ones, may give less clue to origin as inferior detachment may be produced from either inferior or superior breaks. Central vision will be severely impaired when the macula detaches.

The density of field defect varies with the SRF depth, the deeper the fluid the denser the scotoma. Posture may affect SRF depth, e.g. a superior retinal detachment reducing after a period of bed rest may cause diminution or even disappearance of the observed field defect (usually in the morning), only to re-appear again as the patient mobilises. Similarly, in RRD involving the macula, symptoms such as micropsia and metamorphopsia may be absent in the morning, but may progressively appear during the day as the patient mobilises.

Field defects
● Inferior defects indicate an RRD has started superiorly
● Superior defects do not indicate an RRD has started inferiorly
● Inferior defects are noticed early
● Superior field defects are noticed late
● Intensity of field defects varies with the depth of SRF

Other Symptoms

Classical symptoms may not occur and the detachment is identified in other ways. Reduced visual acuity, as the only signpost of RRD, arises in the following ways:

● Macular detachment
● Opacity obscuring RRD
● Anterior uveitis

Macular Detachment

Insidious detachment of the macula is particularly likely to occur with:

- Inferior breaks (e.g. retinal dialysis)
- Pseudophakic detachments. Reduced central vision is often the commonest mode of presentation. Even this may not be taken seriously by patients who have been warned to expect reduction of vision due to capsular thickening.
- Breaks at the posterior pole (e.g. a macular break)

Opacities Obscuring RRD

- Vitreous haemorrhage. Severe vitreous haemorrhage caused by retinal break formation may depress central vision even if retinal detachment is peripheral.
- Inflammation.

Reduced VA and RRD

- Macular detachment:
  SRF spread from periphery
  SRF originates from break at posterior pole
- Macula not detached:
  opacities in media

Anterior Uveitis

Anterior uveitis may complicate RRD and reduce central vision. Flare and cells with fibrinous exudate may be found in the anterior chamber and posterior synechiae form. With posterior uveitis inflam-matory debris in the vitreous body may obscure RRD.

Asymptomatic Detachments

Asymptomatic detachment without depression of central vision are usually detected during routine ophthalmoscopy on patients in whom the examiner has a high index of suspicion of retinal disease, e.g. in the second eye of a patient with RRD or following trauma.

Clinical Summary Points

- Flashes of light and floaters in patients of over 40 years of age indicate vitreous detachment and require urgent examination (within 24 hours) to exclude retinal breaks and early RRD.
- Flashes of light combined with floaters are more likely to be associated with break formation than floaters alone.
- If PVD is complicated by vitreous haemorrhage then risk of retinal break is higher.
- Pigment in the retrolenticular space strongly suggests a retinal break with or without RRD.
- A progressive field defect indicates RRD. Inferior field defects are of localising value as to the site of origin of the RRD, superior field defects are not.
- RRD should be excluded in all cases of reduced visual acuity.
- RRD should be excluded in all cases of anterior uveitis.
- Asymptomatic RRD should be excluded in high-risk cases.

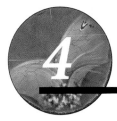

4 Rhegmatogenous Retinal Detachment: Details of Examination

Pre-operative examination enables:

- Assessment of the need for any pre-surgical treatment.
- Consideration of the differential diagnosis of RRD.
- A decision to be made about the choice of surgical procedures and the need or not for prophylactic treatment.
- Informed discussion with the patient (and/ or relatives).

The initial examination is that of the anterior segment and is conducted at the slit-lamp. This is followed by examination of the posterior segment by indirect ophthalmoscopy with scleral depression. This in turn is followed by a further visit to the slit-lamp for contact and non-contact lens examination.

Examination of the Anterior Segment and Vitreous

Examination of the cornea, anterior chamber, lens–iris diaphragm, retrolental space and anterior vitreous is made during the first visit to the slit-lamp. The cornea and anterior chamber (including measurement of intraocular pressure) should be made prior to dilatation of the pupils. All other aspects of the examination including, lens, retrolental space, anterior vitreous and retina should be made after full dilatation of the pupils (cyclopentolate 1% and phenylephrine 10% remains the best combination). Corneal opacities occasionally interfere with the view of the fundus; these include opacities secondary to corneal disease (e.g. trachoma), corneal oedema secondary to endothelial dysfunction or raised intraocular pressure, or corneal sutures following recent repair of injury or corneal grafting. It is rare for opacities to be of such severity that corneal grafting either prior to vitreoretinal surgery or as a combined procedure is necessary.

Anterior Chamber

Typically, intraocular pressure is lower in eyes with retinal detachment, but sometimes raised intraocular pressure may be found. This indicates either an underlying glaucomatous state (e.g. chronic simple glaucoma) or is related to the detachment itself, when it is usually secondary to anterior uveitis. In the latter cases reattachment of the retina results in spontaneous lowering of the intraocular pressure. If intraocular pressure is raised prior to surgery, medical treatment in the form of timolol or diamox is necessary.

Uveitis

Anterior uveitis is sometimes quite brisk and may require medication in the form of local steroids to reduce anterior chamber activity prior to surgery.

The Iris

If pupillary dilatation to a level of approximately 3–4 mm is not achieved then difficulty will be found in examining the peripheral retina. The cause of failure of pupillary dilatation may be physiological, e.g. in heavily melanotic irides or one of a variety of pathological states such as diabetes, intracapsular aphakia (particularly if the surgery has been complicated by vitreous loss), iris clip intraocular lenses, Marfan's syndrome or the prolonged use of miotics for the treatment of chronic simple glaucoma.

The Lens and Capsules

Position of Lens, Pseudophakia and the Lens Capsules

If the crystalline lens is subluxated or even dislocated, as may be found in Marfan's syndrome or following trauma, observation of the peripheral fundus is more difficult. The presence of intraocular lenses may make examination of the retina more difficult, not only because of less satisfactory pupillary dilatation but also because of distortion of the retinal view and annoying reflexes from their surface. If the extracapsular method of cataract surgery has been used thickening of either posterior or anterior capsule may add to the difficulty in visualisation of the peripheral fundus, (Fig. 4.1) a difficulty that is compounded by Elschnig pearl formation.

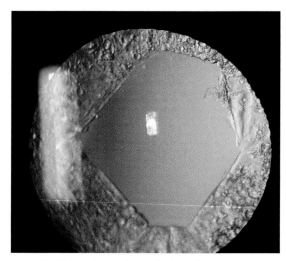

Fig. 4.1. Posterior capsular opacification with capsulotomy.

Lens Opacities

Peripheral cortical opacities frequently interfere with the examination of the fundus, a difficulty that is related to the severity of the lens opacity.

Retrolental Space

Pigment

The retrolental space and vitreous will usually be found to contain pigment granules (tobacco dusting) when a retinal detachment is present (the Schaffer sign) (Fig. 4.2). Exceptions to this may be cases of retinal dialysis or detachments that have complicated retinoschisis when PVD is poorly developed. The pigment is derived from pigment epithelium and arrives by traversing the vitreous cavity via the retinal breaks. This is a very useful sign to indicate the presence of retinal breaks or retinal detachment.

Red Cells

Red cells in the retrolental space and anterior vitreous are found when there has been vitreous haemorrhage. In severe cases pooling of blood in a hyphaema-like arrangement is found in the space

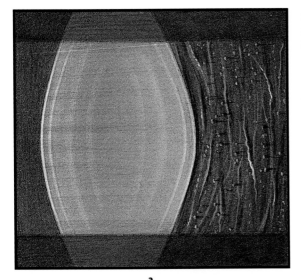

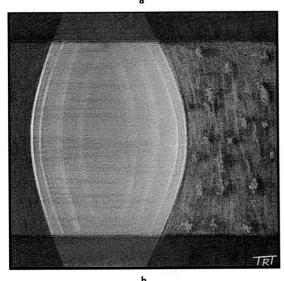

Fig. 4.2. a Pigment granules in the anterior gel in fresh retinal detachment; **b** Pigment clumping in retinal detachment complicated by PVR.

between the anterior hyaloid and the posterior lens capsule.

White Cells

A few white cells may be found in the retrolental space or anterior vitreous of patients with RRD. If marked vitritis is present accumulation of inflam-

matory cells may contribute to both vitreous degeneration and collapse, and enhance the formation and development of periretinal membranes.

Anterior Vitreous

Although examination of the mid and posterior vitreous cavity is best performed with a lens, the anterior third of the vitreous gel may be examined at this stage. This examination is enhanced by making use of eye movement. The patient is asked to look up and then down and then returning the position of gaze to the mid-line. This movement of the eye sets the gel in movement, thereby facilitating interpretation of the physical signs. Normal vitreous gel appears to have a delicate ribbon-like structure, a characteristic feature being its vigorous mobility, which is easily seen. When the vitreous degenerates, this ribbon-like structure is lost and the vitreous substance has a more fibrillary appearance and is less compact in structure. If the posterior vitreous detachment has been complete the posterior hyaloid face is easily seen and with it the area from which the vitreous has detached from the disc (Weiss's ring). However, in the absence of such obvious posterior vitreous detachment it is often difficult to be certain about vitreous detachments in both attached and detached retina. Not infrequently, interpretation of vitreous signs pre-operatively are proven to be wrong or inaccurate at the time of pars plana vitrectomy. Occasionally the vitreous architecture in young patients is completely abnormal (e.g. in Stickler's Syndrome) where the normal characteristics of vitreous gel are absent and indeed the gel has an optically empty appearance.

Proliferative Vitreoretinopathy (PVR)

Involvement of the gel in the process of PVR varies considerably. Sometimes the gel is relatively spared whereas in others it may be extensively affected. If so its normal gel-like structure collapses as does its normal mobility and the gel becomes infiltrated by semi-transparent fibrotic strands which are usually extensively laden with pigment. These may be arranged in large clumps in the vitreous cavity and on the pre-retinal surface or in a string-like fashion.

Examination of Detached Retina

The examination of the detached retina is carried out with indirect ophthalmoscopy and scleral depression. However, these observations need to be confirmed and augmented by returning the patient to the slit lamp for non-contact and or contact lens examination. The latter examination is particularly for the study of the macula, and for providing a magnified view of retinal details, and for study of particular aspects of the vitreoretinal relationship. The most important features concern the macula, the SRF, the breaks, and PVR. On some occasions there may be additional special features such as signs of longstanding detachment, previous surgery, haemorrhage, and choroidal detachment.

The Macula

Macular Detachment

Although reduction of central vision may be caused by overhanging bullous retinal detachment, or opacities in the media, profound reduction of central vision is usually explained by involvement of the macula in the process of RRD.

Macula involvement is important:

1. To determine the urgency of the procedure; thus cases of recent RRD without macula detachment should be operated on as soon as possible to stop the macula detaching.
2. If the macula has been detached the patient has to be warned about the chances of depression of central vision following successful anatomical reattachment. Where the macula has been detached for less than 2 weeks 80% will achieve a central vision of 6/18 or better (6/18 represents about 40% of normal acuity). The longer the macula is detached the worse will be the recovery of central vision.

Other Macular Pathology

Careful examination of the macula with hand held aspheric or contact lenses will reveal the presence of:

● Macular pucker
● Macular holes
● Cystic changes.

All these changes will indicate that the restoration of central vision following vitreoretinal surgery may be less favourable than usual.

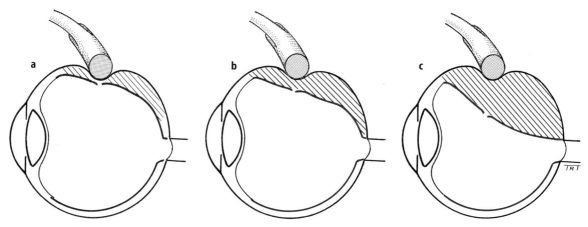

Fig. 4.3. Estimation of subretinal depth under break at pre-operative scleral depression. **a** Break easily closed; **b** some intervening SRF between break and pigment epithelium; **c** deep SRF between pigment epithelium and break.

Subretinal Fluid

The study of the SRF is of importance in the pre-operative assessment process (1) because distribution of SRF conforms with the position of the retinal break; and (2) because of the depth of SRF.

- SRF under the retinal break. The depth of SRF between the break(s) and the pigment epithelium is an important facet of the pre-operative examination. This depth can be roughly estimated when the scleral depressor is applied pre-operatively under the retinal break. If the break can be closed easily then the non-drainage operation will be preferred. However, if fluid between break and pigment epithelium is very deep then non-drainage is difficult as localisation of break and application of retinopexy is more complex (Fig. 4.3).
- Site of deep SRF. If an operation is planned at which SRF is to be drained, it is important to note the position of deep SRF as this area will be chosen as the site for drainage. This observation must be checked at the time of surgery due to the risk of redistribution of fluid after the initial examination has been made.
- Response to bed-rest. On some occasions, bed-rest may be selected to allow flattening of the retina prior to surgery.
- Shift of SRF (see Chap. 3).

Examination of the Retinal Breaks

Successful retinal surgery depends upon the detection and closure of all retinal breaks present in detached retina. The ease of detection and closure of these breaks will be an important factor in defining the complexity of the case, e.g. small breaks are difficult to find but easy to close, and large ones easy to find but difficult to close. Thus a careful pre-operative examination, which should be thorough and unhurried, to note all breaks is fundamental. The position and features of the retinal breaks is one of the most important factors in deciding the type of operation required to achieve reattachment.

The following are the more important features to be noted about retinal breaks:

- Type. The description of breaks according to their shape, size and position has already been discussed (Chap. 3).
- Relationship to each other. When breaks are multiple (about 50% of cases) buckling becomes more difficult. In cases when there is more than one break the majority (60%) are situated within one quadrant of each other. In other cases breaks may not only be widely separated, but be of different sizes and radial orientation making the buckling process more complex.

Relationship to Anatomical Landmarks

Charting of the position of the retinal breaks is made with reference to convenient anatomical landmarks; thus the site of the long ciliary bundles will indicate whether the breaks are in the upper or lower half of the retina, and further orientation is achieved by an imaginary line drawn vertically through the disc dividing the retina into temporal and nasal halves. The twelve o'clock position being referred to as immediately above the disc and the six o'clock immediately below it. The posterior extremity of the breaks is estimated by noting their relationship to the seen or estimated position of the vortex veins. The position of the breaks then described as equatorial, pre-equatorial, or post-equatorial. Localising of the breaks is aided by noting carefully their relationship to normal (e.g. the retinal vessels) or abnormal features (e.g. pigment clumps) (Fig. 4.4).

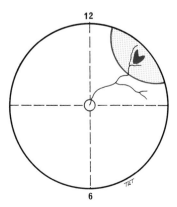

Fig. 4.4. Localisation of retinal breaks.

Summary note

In the examination of the detached retina the most important features are:

- The macula
- The retinal breaks
- SRF details
- PVR and its effect on retina and vitreous

Proliferative Vitreoretinopathy (PVR)

See Chap. 6.

The presence of PVR is important because of its effects on: (1) surgical decision making; and (2) the anatomical and visual prognosis.

Signs of Longstanding RRD

These signs are of importance because (1) long-term macula detachment carries a poor prognosis for restoration of central vision after reattachment; and (2) the relationship of the detachment to alleged or actual trauma in medico-legal cases (i.e. longstanding signs rule out recent trauma as a cause of detachment).

The following changes are found in longstanding RRD; (Fig. 4.5)

- The retina becomes thin and atrophic.
- High-water marks may be seen. These are lines which are pigmented to a varying degree and form in flat retina ahead of an advancing wall of SRF and are often seen in longstanding RRD. These water marks take at least 3 months to form

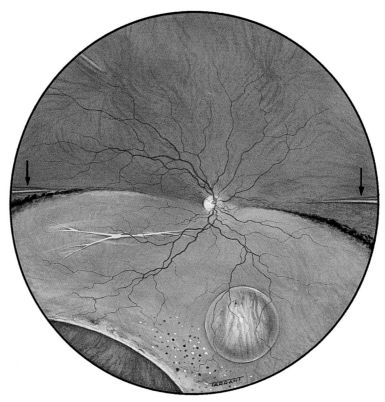

Fig. 4.5. Longstanding retinal detachment. High-water marks are present below the long ciliary bundles. Retro-retinal strands are seen and secondary intraretinal cyst formation has occurred. Whitish and pigmented vitreous opacities are seen overlying a retinal dialysis.

following retinal detachment. Sequential levels of water marks may be found if there has been slow advance of the detachment edge. Thus, demarcation lines do not offer complete protection against further detachment of retina, but may contribute to slower progression and sometimes SRF may have retreated from a previous high-water marks.

- Retro-retinal strands. In longstanding retinal detachment an interlacing network of retro-retinal white lines may be seen. Although, these structures (a form of PVR) are relatively benign in behaviour and rarely interfere with reattachment, they may occasionally be severe enough to warrant surgical removal.
- Intra-retinal Cysts. Cystic spaces large enough to be clinically obvious may develop in the outer plexiform layer of the retina when retinal detachment has been longstanding (at least 1 year). They are of striking ophthalmological appearance, but do not pose any particular problem to reattachment of the retina disappearing spontaneously in the post-operative period after the break has been closed. They may occasionally interfere with break closure if situated in the immediate vicinity of a break.
- Peripheral retinal vessels may develop telangiectatic formations or tuft like projections.

> The features of long-standing RRD are:
> - Thin retina
> - High-water marks
> - Retro-retinal strands
> - Intraretinal cysts

Previous Surgery

Cases that have had previous operations pose problems because (1) examination is more difficult; and (2) the surgical approach may need to be modified. Examination is made more difficult because:

1. Buckles may interfere with adequate scleral depression especially if the eye is tender and photophobic. Greater reliance will have to be placed therefore on contact and non-contact lens examination.

2. Break detection is more difficult because:
   - The white reflex from previous retinopexy reduces contrast between neuro-epithelium and pigment epithelium.
   - Vitreous haze (due to breakdown of the blood–retina barrier) tends to become more pronounced.
   - Retinal adhesion at points of previous retinopexy makes the retinal contours more difficult to interpret and therefore they become a less reliable indicator of break position.

Haemorrhage

Retinal

Small round haemorrhages are often found in the vicinity of retinal breaks in cases of fresh retinal detachment and are produced as a result of PVD. They are clinically insignificant, but their presence may serve as a useful signpost in aiding the detection of breaks. Small haemorrhages are sometimes found in longstanding retinal detachments where they are often thinly scattered in the periphery of the detached retina.

Vitreous

Some degree of spontaneous vitreous haemorrhage is commonly found in cases of retinal detachment and is usually associated with a rupture of a blood vessel during the development of a retinal break (Fig. 4.6).

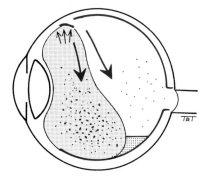

Fig. 4.6. Vitreous haemorrhage from retinal break formation. Blood from a retinal tear (small arrows) spreads either into the retro-gel compartment or into the gel itself.

Haemorrhage occurs most frequently from an upper half retinal tear and descends by gravity down the back of the posterior hyaloid face or passes into the vitreous gel. A combination is often seen (Fig. 4.7).

Retrovitreal haemorrhage may be found in the inferior retina piled up on the back of the posterior hyaloid face at its juncture with the retina. In the aphakic or pseudophakic eye, blood may pass into the anterior chamber to cause hyphaema, and the egress of blood via the angle will improve the rate of clearance from the eye. The behaviour and spread of vitreous haemorrhage following clotting and lysis depends mainly on the extent of the haemorrhage and the state of the vitreous gel. In the young eye, intra-vitreal or pre-retinal collections of blood take weeks or months to clear, but do so more readily in the highly myopic with degenerate vitreous or in the vitrectomised eye. Blood in the vitreous cavity is metabolised slowly, and evidence of old haemorrhage is provided by the presence of a whitish coagulum that is usually found in the inferior gel.

In the majority of cases haemorrhage is slight and is of little clinical significance, but if severe may:

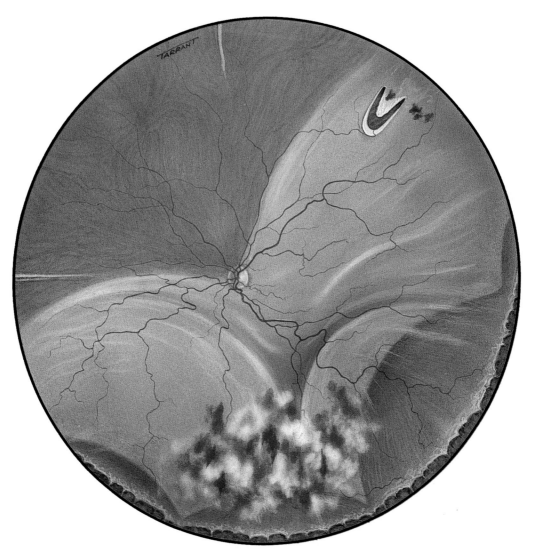

Fig. 4.7. Retinal detachment. Fresh ultrasound blood in seen in the vitreous. Choroidal detachment is present.

- Obscure the view of the retina either partially or completely.
- Promote PVR.
- Increase the risk of secondary uveitis and glaucoma due to diffusion of blood cells into the anterior chamber.

Causes of vitreous haemorrhage

- PVD – uncomplicated
- Retinal break
- Trauma
- Previous surgery
- Proliferative retinopathies
- Terson's syndrome

Choroidal

Choroidal haemorrhage is either secondary to trauma or as an operative complication of vitreo-retinal surgery.

Choroidal Detachment

Serous choroidal detachments are occasionally found pre-operatively in eyes with retinal detachments (4.5% in one series). They are particularly associated with RRD and high myopia. They are recognised by their characteristic dark rounded outlines seen through the retinal detachment (Fig. 4.7). They may be localised or annular in extent and are identical in appearance to the choroidal detachments seen following cataract or glaucoma surgery. They are related to the hypotony induced by the process of retinal detachment. The detachments often extend into the vicinity of the ciliary body with reduced aqueous output, but their posterior extension is usually limited by the scleral exit of the vortex veins. If seen pre-operatively and there is no other indication for urgent surgery a period of delay (a week or so) may result in a least partial reabsorption prior to surgery thus making surgery easier. Choroidal detachments are important because:

- There is an increased risk of PVR. This may be partially caused by the inflammation in the eye promoted by choroidal detachment.
- Surgery may be more complex in their presence, e.g. if the choroidal detachment is under a retinal break external cryotherapy will be impossible.

Differential Diagnosis of RRD

Usually the diagnosis of RRD is simple (Table 4.1). The appearance of the detached retina is characterised by undulating folds, loss of choroidal reflex and darkening of retinal vessels and the presence of full-thickness retinal breaks. Occasionally, RRD may be confused with

- Tractional retinal detachment (TRD),
- Retinoschisis
- Non-rhegmatogenous retinal detachment.

RRD and TRD

Contour

Unlike RRD, in TRD the junction between the detached and attached retina is characterised by a

Table 4.1. Differential diagnosis

Feature	Longstanding RRD	TRD	Retinoschisis
Schaffer sign	+ve	–ve	–ve
Breaks	Present	Absent	Outer leaf
Contour	Convex	Concave	Convex
High-water marks	Present	Present (maybe)	Absent
Position in fundus	Extends to ora	Localised	Extends to ora
Retro-retinal strands	Present (usually)	Present (maybe)	Absent
Other eye involvement	Unusual	Unusual (maybe)	Usual
Unaffected Retina	Normal	May reflect cause of TRD – e.g. diabetes	Normal

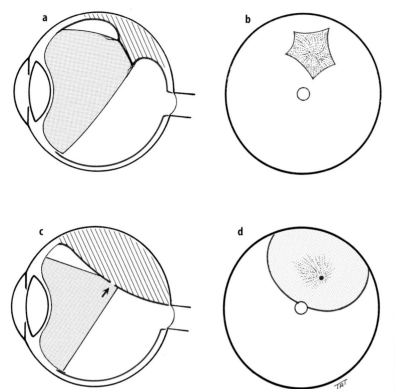

Fig. 4.8. (**a** and **b**) Traction retinal detachment (TRD). The TRD is concave towards the vitreous cavity and also towards attached retina; (**c** and **d**) retinal break has complicated the TRD which now has a rhegmatogenous element and becomes convex towards the vitreous cavity and towards attached retina.

concave border towards flat retina and in TRD the retina is also concave towards the vitreous cavity (Fig. 4.8).

Breaks

In TRD full-thickness retinal breaks are absent.

RRD and Retinoschisis

In longstanding RRD the retinal texture appears thinner and more atrophic and loses the typical appearance of freshly detached retina. It can therefore come to resemble the appearance of retinoschisis. However, it is distinguished by the following:

- Demarcation line or secondary retinal cysts are not seen in retinoschisis
- Full-thickness breaks are not seen in retinoschisis

- Retinoschisis is usually bilateral, asymptomatic with no premonitory signs or visual loss.

RRD and Non-Rhegmatogenous RD

There is usually little difficulty in distinguishing these two conditions. RRD is characterised by the presence of full-thickness breaks and non-rhegmatogenous RD by the presence of inferior shifting SRF (e.g. in Harada's disease or uveal effusion syndrome). However, if retinal detachment is unilateral and breaks are not seen then the distinction between the two conditions is less certain, particularly if there are no other signs of ocular disease which might produce non-rhegmatogenous retinal detachment (e.g. malignant melanoma or inflammatory changes within the vitreous as in scleritis). In cases of diagnostic difficulty ultrasonography (showing a thickened sclera in scleritis) and fluorescein angiography (showing pigment epithelial disturbance) may be useful additional investigations.

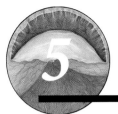

5 Rhegmatogenous Retinal Detachment: Features of Special Types

involved in the mechanism of dialysis production and is only found if it occurs spontaneously at a later date. The vitreous base remains attached to the posterior edge of the dialysis, an attachment that results in some degree of immobility of the break (Fig. 5.1).

Retinal dialysis is commonly associated with contusive trauma and therefore occurs more commonly in young men. If a dialysis is found in the upper nasal quadrant of the retina this is pathognomonic of contusive injury to the eye. However, the commonest site of a dialysis is the lower temporal quadrant where the role of trauma is much less obvious. It is not clear why this site is prone to the development of this type of retinal break. Trauma certainly plays a part in some of these cases, but occasionally

RRD – Features of Special Types

- Dialysis
- Giant break
- Retinoschisis
- Cataract surgery
- Features suggesting a poor prognosis

Cases may be described as special either because they have distinctive or unusual clinical features or because they have appearances suggesting a poorer prognosis than usual due to anticipated difficulties in reattachment. These detachments may have

- Unusual breaks
- RRD associated with other posterior segment disorders
- RRD after cataract surgery
- Additional features of RRD suggesting a poor prognosis.

Unusual Breaks

These are retinal dialyses, giant breaks, macular and other breaks at the posterior pole.

Retinal Dialysis

Dialysis is the term applied to breaks at the ora serrata. Posterior vitreous detachment is not

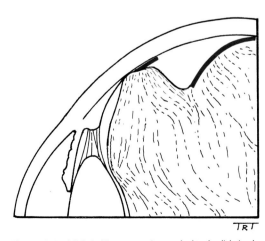

Fig. 5.1. Retinal dialysis. Vitreous remains attached to the dialysis edge.

the condition is found to be bilateral (approximately 5%), indicating that the ora serrata may have an underlying weakness in the lower temporal quadrant. As well as in contusive injury, dialysis may also occur in penetrating injury. In such cases it is usually found close to the site of penetration, be this with a foreign body or occasionally in association with instrumentation introduced through sclerotomy sites at pars plana vitrectomy (PPV).

> Upper nasal dialysis is pathognomonic of trauma

Clinical Features

- The premonitory symptoms of vitreous detachment do not occur and the condition usually presents only when visual acuity is noticed as reduced or discovered in the course of an examination.
- In inferior dialysis, accumulation of SRF is slow so that at the time of presentation the macula is detached in the large majority of cases (85%). As time progresses signs of longstanding detachment appear (see Chap. 4 and Fig. 4.5).
- In the majority of cases the eyes are emmetropic.

Break Features

When the dialysis is fresh the break may be slit-like and difficult to detect, requiring gentle peripheral scleral depression. Dialyses may be multiple and if so are usually situated in the same quadrant of the retina separated by small bridges of retinal tissue. Giant dialysis (extending for more than one quadrant) is exceptionally rare. If longstanding the presence of the dialysis is often signposted by characteristic whitish opacities and pigment collections in the vitreous overlying the dialysis (Chiggy's dots). With age the dialysis becomes easier to see, as it becomes somewhat retracted.

Progression

With inferior dialyses it is unusual for the SRF to rise much higher than the midline.

PVR

The presence of PVR is usually limited to sub-retinal strand formation and pre-retinal membrane formation is usually absent.

Surgery

RRD secondary to dialysis responds readily to conventional buckling surgery. Reattachment is usually achieved, but return of central vision fol-lowing longstanding detachment of the macula is usually disappointing.

Retinal dialysis
• Young patients   • Premonitory symptoms of flashes and floaters are absent   • May be associated with contusive or perforating trauma   • Progression is insidious   • Macula usually detached at presentation   • Detection requires careful scleral indentation.   • High-water marks and secondary intra-retinal cysts may be found   • Responds favourably to conventional surgery, but visual results are often poor

Giant Breaks

Giant breaks are defined as those that extend for 90° or more of the retinal circumstances.

Although these cases are rare (approximately 1% of most retinal detachments series) they are important because they raise particular problems in management due to difficulties in reattachment. Most cases arise spontaneously following PVD although they may occur following either penetrating or contusive trauma (including cataract surgery complicated by vitreous loss and the manipulation of the vitreous resulting in direct vitreo-retinal traction). Some are associated with congenital abnormalities (e.g. Stickler's syndrome). The mechanism by which giant breaks are formed is poorly understood.

Clinical Features

The average age of this group is lower than that in the detachment population as a whole and the male sex is favoured. There is a greater tendency to myopia. The breaks arise in the pre-equatorial region (the temporal side being more affected than the nasal) from retina that had no obvious abnormality. The upper half of the retina is much more likely to be affected than the lower. It is rare for lattice degeneration to be found (except in cases of Stickler's Syndrome where extensive lattice changes may be found), but areas of white without pressure may be seen both in the affected and fellow eye. In non-traumatic cases the eventual incidence of bilaterality is approximately 50%. In addition to the usual symptoms of posterior vitreous detachment the movement of the mobile posterior flap of a giant break may produce the unusual symptom of a dense moving curtain passing in front of the eye as it interferes with central vision.

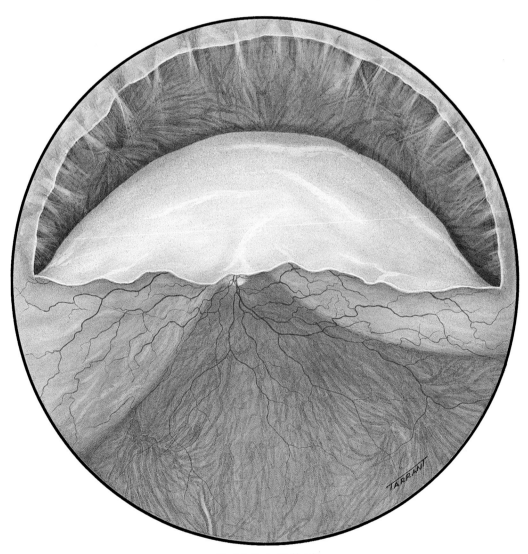

Fig. 5.2. Giant retinal break.

Break Features

In a giant retinal break the posterior hyaloid is firmly attached to the anterior flap of the break, allowing independent mobility of the posterior flap of the break (Figs. 5.2, 5.3). Attachment of vitreous usually produces quite substantial elevation of the anterior post-oral retina. Satellite tears are often found in association with the extremities of the giant break at the same circumferential level and occasionally they are quite numerous. In giant retinal dialysis (exceptionally rare) vitreous remains attached to the posterior edge of the retina. In a giant break the movement of the posterior flap is variable and although tending to stay in situ initially will usually subsequently flap back over so that the back of the neuro-epithelium is viewed on ophthalmoscopy.

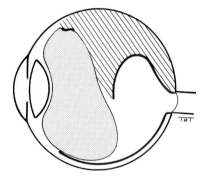

Fig. 5.3. There is no vitreous attachment to the posterior edge of the break which is freely mobile.

Progression of RRD

Surprisingly in giant breaks of recent onset retinal detachment itself may be limited, but eventually the retina becomes totally detached.

PVR

Giant breaks have a particular tendency to form peri-retinal membranes presumably due to the easy access of pigment epithelium to the pre-retinal surface. These membranes eventually limit the movement of the flap which becomes progressively more immobilised. The flap itself will tend to roll up and become fixed in a retroverted position and eventually incorporated into dense fibrous tissue.

Surgery

The surgery of giant breaks is difficult and requires PPV.

Family History

In cases of Stickler's syndrome other members of the family should be examined as there is a strong family history in this condition.

Giant retinal breaks
• Giant breaks are rare
• They usually arise spontaneously
• The vitreous is attached to the anterior edge of the break
• The posterior flap of retina is initially freely mobile
• Satellite breaks are common
• PVR appears rapidly
• Surgery is difficult and requires PPV

Macular Breaks

Although rare, macular breaks associated with RRD are of importance because of the difficulty that they pose in clinical management. These breaks are almost invariably round holes. Senile macular holes of a degenerative nature in a non-myopic eye do not progress to RRD (see Chap. 19).

Macular breaks may be found in association with RRD in the following ways (Fig. 5.4):

1. High myopia. The macular holes in these cases are responsible for the production of the RRD. Slit-lamp biomicroscopy is required to see these breaks which are poorly contrasted with the underlying white reflex from choroido-retinal atrophy which is invariably present. The role of vitreous traction is uncertain, but focal vitreo-retinal traction on the break is rarely seen. Posterior staphyloma is usually present. SRF accumulates progressively and often quite slowly from the posterior pole, but eventually spreads to involve peripheral retina. The premonitory symptoms of retinal detachment are usually absent. Patients usually notice reduction of central vision as the presenting symptom.

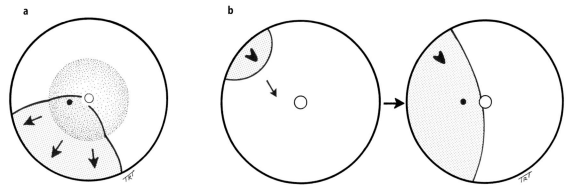

Fig. 5.4. **a** The macular hole is the primary cause of RRD; **b** The macular hole is secondary to peripheral RRD.

Surgery: PPV is usually necessary to treat these cases.

2. Macular holes occasionally form as a secondary effect of the advancing wall of subretinal fluid, arriving at the macula from the extension of a peripheral retinal detachment from a peripheral break. The reason why secondary macular holes may form in this way is very poorly understood. The restoration of central vision following reattachment is prejudiced by their presence.

Surgery: needs only to concentrate on closure of the peripheral break.

Other Breaks at the Posterior Pole

Breaks other than at the macula are unusual but may be found:

- As small para-vascular slits in the highly myopic eye
- Large tears following acute posterior vitreous detachment in the contused eye
- Small iatrogenic perforations may be found in the posterior pole because of accidental damage caused by perforation of the globe as a consequence of local anaesthetic blocks.

Surgery: PPV is needed.

RRD and Other Posterior Segment Disorders

- RRD and choroidal detachment (see Chap. 4)
- RRD and retinoschisis
- RRD and TRD
- RRD and coloboma
- RRD and inflammation

Retinoschisis and Retinal Detachment

RRD complicating retinoschisis is rare. If RRD occurs then breaks are found in both inner and outer layers of the retinoschisis cavity. Inner leaf breaks (connecting the schisis cavity with the vitreous compartment) are round holes and difficult to find. Outer leaf breaks connecting the schisis cavity to the subretinal space may vary substantially in size and can be large and oval or kidney-shaped, often with a rather ill-defined rolled posterior border (Fig. 5.5). Signs of retinoschisis are usually found in the other eye. Occasionally, retinoschisis may be found as an incidental feature in an eye with retinal detachment where a break arises quite separately from the area of schisis. In these cases, the retinal detachment can be treated ignoring the schisis.

Surgery: these cases are usually treated by conventional surgery with drainage of subretinal fluid and buckling to close both inner and outer leaf

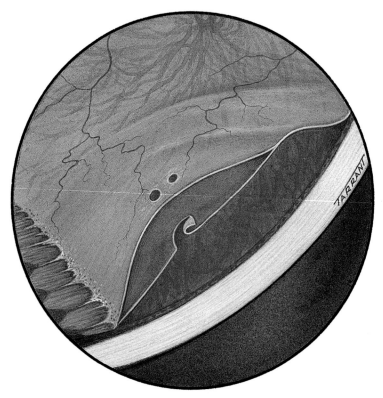

Fig. 5.5. Retinoschisis complicated by RRD. Inner and outer leaf breaks are seen.

breaks. If this is not possible then PPV may be needed. This may be difficult as posterior vitreous detachment is often poorly developed.

RRD Secondary to TRD

In a small proportion of patients with TRD complicating vaso-proliferative retinopathy of which diabetes is by far the most common (others include branch vein occlusion, HbSc disease and inflammatory retinopathies), a full-thickness break may be produced as a consequence of vitreo-retinal traction. These breaks are usually found in close proximity to the fibrotic component of the neovascular complex and therefore most often found in the posterior retina. Reduction of vision is the commonest presenting feature due to detachment of the macula; other premonitory symptoms do not occur (see Chap. 3).

Surgery: these cases almost invariably require PPV to achieve relief of vitreo-retinal traction and internal closure of the retinal breaks.

RRD and Coloboma

Retinal detachment is sometimes seen in uveal colobomata and may be of two main types:

1. The detachment arises from breaks quite separate from the coloboma itself, in which case the detachment can be managed without regard to the coloboma.
2. The detachment appears to have arisen from breaks in the coloboma. These breaks are difficult to find and these cases are usually treated with PPV.

RRD Secondary to Inflammatory Disease

Breaks leading to RRD may be produced in inflammatory ocular disease in a variety of ways:

- Infiltration of white cells into the vitreous may cause degeneration and collapse with PVD and retinal break formation. This is an unusual complication of uveitis.

  Surgery: if the retinal view is good and the breaks can be detected then conventional retinal surgery may be used. If the view is poor due to vitreous opacities, then PPV will be needed.

- Breaks may be produced by contraction of focal areas of inflammatory fibrotic tissue (e.g. on the edge of a toxocara scar in the retinal periphery).

  Surgery: it is often difficult to find these breaks and PPV will usually be necessary.

- RRD may be secondary to TRD in inflammatory vaso-proliferative disease (e.g. sarcoidosis).

  Surgery: PPV.

- Retina may be directly weakened by inflammation (e.g. acute retinal necrosis, and cytomegalovirus retinitis) resulting in melting of retinal tissue and break formation. The latter may be exacerbated by vitreous detachment induced by inflammation.

  Surgery: PPV.

Clinical Features of Retinal Detachment after Cataract Surgery

The usual interval between cataract extraction and retinal detachment is approximately 1 year. This interval is considerably shortened if vitreous has been lost at the time of surgery and greatly lengthened in the case of retinal detachment following congenital cataract surgery where the interval may be 15–20 years. Total retinal detachment appears to occur more readily than in the phakic eye and macular detachment is disappointingly common (about 85% of cases). There is an increased tendency for retinal breaks to be multiple.

Special problems of RRD management after cataract surgery are:

- Break detection. A reduced view is caused by lens or capsular remnants and difficulty with pupillary dilatation, (e.g. caused by posterior synechiae or pupil capture). These difficulties are compounded by awkward reflexes from the intraocular lens.

- Peroperative difficulties (see Chap. 15). These include difficulty in visualisation, instability of the intraocular lens, (with a risk of dislocation and haemorrhage into the anterior chamber) and difficulties with gas injection into the eye, e.g. gas may enter the anterior chamber (see Chap. 15).

Surgery

If the retinal view is good and breaks can be found then the detachment may be treated in exactly the same way as phakic eyes (see Chap. 10). In the event of obscuration of the retinal view, PPV is necessary and is useful in a substantial proportion of pseudophakic cases, particularly as the main complication of PPV (i.e. the production of a lens opacity) cannot occur.

Features of RRD Suggesting a Poor Prognosis

These are the clinical signs that indicate successful reattachment will be difficult and that visual expectations are reduced:

- Threatened PVR
- Established PVR (see Chap. 6)

Threatened PVR

PVR is not established, but risk factors for its development are present and these include:

- Difficult breaks. Breaks may be described as difficult either when they are going to be a problem to close because of their size (a giant break is an extreme example), because of their position (posterior breaks are difficult to get at), because of a complex arrangement (breaks widely scattered and arranged at different antero-posterior location) or because they are poorly seen. If breaks are not closed failure will occur and the appearance of PVR promoted.

- Uveitis
- Haemorrhage (vitreous and choroid).
- Choroidal detachments.
- Perforating injuries.
- Combined RRD and TRD
- Failed surgery

Nothing is more likely to promote failure than a poorly conceived surgical approach. If breaks are not closed and retina remains or becomes re-detached then the inflammation induced by the various surgical moves (e.g. cryotherapy, SRF drainage, vitreous gases) will contribute to the production of PVR.

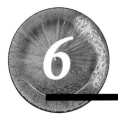

6 Proliferative Vitreo-retinopathy (PVR)

PVR is the growth of fibrocellular tissue on the surface of the retina and the vitreo-retinal interface. It is a modified form of wound healing initiated by retinal breaks and usually resolves by prompt reattachment of the retina.

Pathobiology

The biological response to retinal detachments involves the following:

- Initial injury: inflammatory response associated with breakdown of blood ocular barrier.
- Cellular response: formation of simple epiretinal membranes and complex epiretinal membranes.
- Role of cytokines and matricellular proteins
- Re-modelling and contraction of the extra-cellular matrix
- Resolution.

Initial Injury

The PVR process can be considered as a modified wound healing process which is initiated by injury. In the case of the retina the injury begins with the formation of the retinal break associated with varying amounts of haemorrhage from broken blood vessels. The internal limiting lamina of the retina is breached. Having lost its apposition to the neuro-sensory retina, the cells of the retinal pigment epithelium are liberated and gain access to the vitreous cavity via the break. The early response is one of inflammation accompanied by the breakdown of the blood–retina barrier. Macrophages (derived from blood monocytes and retinal neural elements) and lymphocytes infiltrate the vitreous cavity. The breakdown of the blood–ocular barrier permits fibrin and clotting cascade proteins to enter the vitreous cavity.

Cellular Response and the Formation of Simple Epiretinal Membranes

The break in the internal limiting lamina stimulates glial cells to migrate to the inner retina surface. The initial simple epiretinal membranes that form are

> Break closure and retinal reattachment prevents PVR onset or halts progression

made up of glial elements on the surface of the retina. Further recruitment of retinal pigment epithelial and other cells contributes to the formation of complex epiretinal membranes. As with any wound healing process, cytokines play a vital role in cell-to-cell interactions including recruitment, proliferation, secretion of extracellular matrix, adhesion and migration.

Role of Cytokines and Matricellular Proteins

Cytokines are small polypeptides or glycoproteins and they bind to specific receptors on cell surfaces. They act as chemical mediators between different cell types. Important cytokines include growth factors, e.g. transforming growth factor-β, fibroblast growth factors, platelet-derived growth factor and the interleukins (I, II and VI). Other cytokines which have been demonstrated to play a role in PVR include cell adhesion molecules and tissue necrotic factors. Larger proteins such as fibronectin and fibrin degregation product are strongly chemotatic and may perform an important function in cellular recruitment.

The cellular component of complex epiretinal membranes is mixed. Epiretinal membranes vary greatly in the degree of cellularity with younger membranes being more cellular. Immunological staining has identified a proportion of the cells being of retinal pigment epithelial and glial in origin. There remains a large proportion of fibroblast-like cells the source of which is obscure. All are capable of secretion of extracellular matrix proteins and collagen. These so-called matricellular proteins may form important interactions with the cellular component. Glycoproteins such as thrombospondin, laminin and tenacin interact with the retinal pigment epithelial cells and fibroblast and may modulate their motility.

Re-modelling and Contraction of the Extracellular Matrix

The main fibrous component of epiretinal membranes is type I collagen (with variable amounts of type II, III, IV), laminin and fibronectin. In vitro models have shown that the migration of retinal pigment epithelial cells (and tissue fibroblasts) causes contraction of the collagen fibres. The gathering of the collagen into bundles, secretion and re-modelling leads to the contracted scar tissue. Enzyme systems such as the metallo-proteases secreted by the cells break down the extracellular matrix whilst new collagen is secreted. In vitro, inhibitors of such enzymes stop the motility of retinal pigment epithelial cells in collagen gels and prevent their contracture. As the epiretinal membranes become mature, more collagen is laid down and it becomes relatively hypocellular. Unlike healing in other parts of the body there is usually little or no vascular proliferation.

Resolution

If it is possible to achieve break closure and retinal reattachment, the PVR process often but not invariably enters its resolution phase. The integrity of the blood–ocular barriers is restored and the drive for further cellular proliferation and migration ceases. In some cases, resolution does not occur until there is total retinal detachment with the fibrous contracture leading to the retina adopting a closed funnel configuration and obscuring the optic disc. The precise mechanism by which this resolution process is modulated is unknown.

Clinical Features

Clinically the PVR process is recognised by the following signs:

- Vitreous haze
- Cellular infiltration and relative rigidity of the retina
- Eversion of the edges of the retinal tears
- Diffuse proliferation in the posterior retina
- Focal proliferation manifesting as star folds
- Circumferential contracture along the posterior border of the vitreous base
- Radial contracture of the vitreous base leading to anterior displacement of the retina towards the ciliary process and posterior iris surfaces
- Subretinal fibrosis.

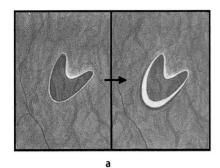 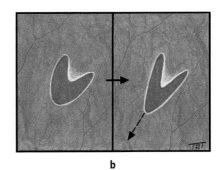

Fig. 6.1. Effect of PVR on breaks: **a** rolling of retinal tear; **b** elongation of tear due to more centrally placed membrane.

The clinical appearances, distribution of PVR, its appearance, rate of progression and response to surgery are still poorly understood. The early stages of PVR are characterised by the presence of vitreous haze. The gel usually shows pigment clumps. There is reduced motility of the gel that can be observed on biomicroscopy and on dynamic B-mode ultrasonography. The edges of retinal tears are rolled and distorted (Fig. 6.1). The operculum of the large retinal tear may be anteverted. Surrounding retinal surfaces appear to be stiffened. Some retinal breaks are obscured by epiretinal membranes. Retinal vessels are drawn into the contracting epicentre of the membrane so that they are straightened centrally and distorted in the immediate vicinity of the membrane. They may also be partially obscured by membrane.

Pre-retinal membranes usually favour the lower half of the retina (probably due to gravitational fallout of cells) and also the anterior third of the retina is more often involved than posterior retina (Fig. 6.2). In moderate PVR, the surface of the retina is wrinkled. Fibrosis may be diffuse and scattered throughout the retina. If focal, the fibrotic areas result in radiating creases in the retina (a starfold; Fig. 6.3). Further contracture of the epiretinal membrane causes the retinal detachment to assume a cone-shaped configuration and eventually, the posterior leaves of the retina may be apposed to form a narrow tube (Fig. 6.4). In advanced PVR, the fibrosis is concentrated in the vicinity of the vitreous base where it gives rise to a purse-string effect. In eyes which had had previous vitrectomy and gas tamponade, the traction process often involves the pars plana and membranes become adherent to the pre-equatorial retina, ciliary processes and sometimes the posterior surface of the iris in aphakic or pseudophakic eyes.

Subretinal membrane is usually associated with longstanding detachments and is found particularly in younger patients and following trauma (Fig. 6.5). If not too extensive it may be ignored as it will not usually interfere with the process of reattachment. However, sometimes they may be very extensive, not only in the peripheral retina, but may affect posterior retina contributing to the funnel effect of retinal detachment (the napkin ring effect around the disc). In these cases surgical removal is necessary.

Predisposing Factors

The following clinical features increase the risk of development of PVR in RRD:

- The presence of large retinal breaks
- The presence of blood in the posterior segment
- Failed surgery (especially if complicated by haemorrhage or excessive cryotherapy)
- Longstanding retinal detachment
- Ocular inflammation

Proliferative vitreoretinopathy is caused by retinal detachment. It is rare for PVR to be present in fresh cases (detachment for less than two weeks). Prompt reattachment by closing all breaks will prevent the appearance of PVR and in cases when PVR is present, but not extensive, reattachment of the retina will result in resolution of the PVR process. Failed surgery however, promotes the onset and progression of PVR making subsequent reattachment very much difficult.

When severe PVR is established, even apparently identifying and closing retinal breaks, and relieving tractional systems upon the retina will not necessarily halt the inexorable march of this process.

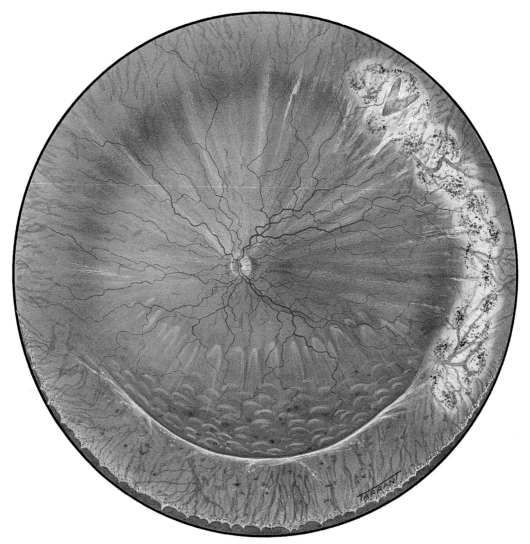

Fig. 6.2. Advanced PVR. Previous retinal surgery has failed. The retina is totally detached, multiple retinal folds are seen in inferior retina with pigment clumps in gel and on the retinal surface. Fibrosis and contraction of the vitreous base pulling ora serrata posteriorly is seen.

Reproliferation and recontraction may reopen apparently closed breaks.

Retinal features and PVR
● Membranes obscure and distort breaks
● Breaks are more difficult to close
● Progression of PVR can reopen closed breaks

Clinical Importance

The presence of PVR is important because it makes retinal reattachment more difficult (the more complex the PVR the more difficult will be the reattachment) and it is also affects the visual result if the macula is involved in the proliferative process. Function is also threatened by the complex surgical moves necessary to achieve reattachment.

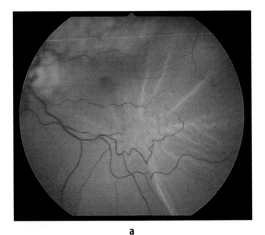

a

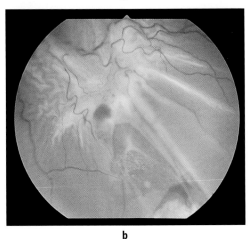

b

Fig. 6.3. a Immature starfold; **b** mature starfold distorting and immobilising a retinal tear.

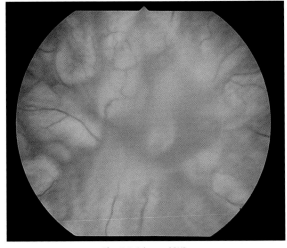

Fig. 6.4. Advanced PVR.

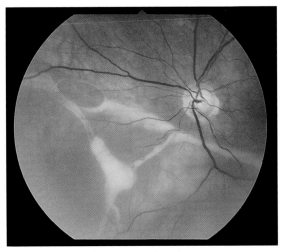

Fig. 6.5. Subretinal membrane.

Classification of PVR

Classification of PVR

Grade A
Vitreous haze, vitreous pigment clumps, pigment clusters on inferior retina

Grade B
Wrinkling of inner retinal surface, retinal stiffness, vessel tortuosity, rolled and irregular edge of retina break, decreased mobility of vitreous

Grade CP 1–12
Posterior to equator :
focal, diffuse, or circumferential full-thickness folds,* subretinal strands*

Grade CA 1–12
Anterior to equator:
focal, diffuse, or circumferential full-thickness folds,* subretinal strands,* anterior displacement,* condensed vitreous with strands

*Expressed in number of clock hours involved)

Grade C PVR		
Type	**Location**	**Features**
1. Focal	Posterior to equator	Starfold posterior to vitreous base
2. Diffuse	Posterior to equator	Confluent starfold posterior to vitreous base
3. Subretinal	Posterior/anterior to equator	Proliferation under the retina: annular strand near disc; linear strands; sheets
4. Circumferential	Anterior to equator	Contraction along posterior edge of vitreous base with central displacement of the retina stretched; posterior retina in radial folds
5. Anterior displacement	Anterior to equator	Vitreous base pulled anteriorly by proliferative tissue; peripheral retinal trough; ciliary process may be stretched, may be covered by membrane; iris may be retracted

This classification is a surgical description of the PVR process at the time of the examination. For example, it will not give any indication as to the onset or rate of progression of the PVR process, nor does it consider retinal breaks. Although the more advanced stages of PVR represent a difficult surgical challenge in terms of overcoming the mechanical problems, it is not a reliable prognostic grading system. Thus some cases of Grade B PVR will progress inexorably and some cases of severe local PVR (following for example trauma) may respond very poorly to surgery, while other very advanced cases may respond well. The grading system should therefore be regarded as providing clinicians with a means of describing the PVR picture. Like retinal drawings for simple retinal detachment, the classification provides a means of documentation. It is important for clinical studies and serves as a shorthand for communication of clinical data.

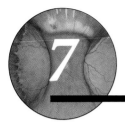

7 Pre-operative Management

The preoperative management of vitreo-retinal cases should include the following:

- Documentation of clinical findings
- Patient information and consent
- Consideration of bed-rest
- General medical treatment
- Treating ocular inflammation and infection.

Clinical Pathway of Care

The use of Clinical Care Pathway is now widely adopted in many branches of medicine. This is a standardised protocol for management of specific conditions and it has many advantages:

1. It provides a checklist all essential elements of the pre-operative and post-operative care

2. It ensures that all important clinical information is properly documented
3. It is an efficient way of communication between doctors, nurses and patients
4. It provides a basis for audit

Documentation

The essential elements of a care pathway for vitreo-retinal surgery should include documentation of the following:

- History and pre-operative findings at presentation
- Diagnosis
- The proposed surgical operation
- Patient/relative counselling
- Informed consent
- Operative details
- Operative complications
- Post-operative management
- Outcome measures

Proper documentation also forms the basis of clinical teaching in research and is an important medico-legal record. In many health services there is a demand for efficiency and a need to audit outcome in order to justify resources.

Counselling Patients

The nature of many vitreo-retinal conditions such as retinal detachment, proliferative diabetic retinopathy and macular holes can be difficult to explain in simple terms to patients. Although explanations should not be unnecessarily complex, patients undergoing vitreo-retinal surgery should have some awareness of the following:

- The nature of the disease and the natural history of the condition
- The success rate of the proposed operation and what success means in terms of both central and peripheral vision
- The possible need for further surgery
- Relevant operative and post-operative complications
- Instructions for post-operative management (such as posture) and a warning about immediate post-operative expectations (e.g. symptoms such as pain, redness and watering of the eye and immediate post-operative visual expectation (may be better or worse)
- Informed consent.

Surgeons may not have the necessary time to impart all the routine information to a patient. Trained nurse practitioners, sometimes with the help of audio-visual aids, can be supportive in this role. The role of counselling is important in cases where patients' co-operation and motivation are required. This particularly applied to the use of internal tamponade and the need for post-operative posturing. Counselling should take into consideration the needs of the individual and the capacity of the patient to absorb and use the information. Some anxious patients need to be reassured by receiving more information whilst others are happier leaving the decisions to the doctors and nurses. In general, it is a good idea to involve relatives, guardians and interpreters in the counselling process unless the patient specifically objects to this. If there are difficult choices to be made (e.g. whether to undergo an operation or not) the burden of the decision should be discussed and shared with other family members.

Bed-Rest

The indications for bed-rest are:

1. To prevent further extension of retinal detachment prior to surgery

2. To reduce the depth of subretinal fluid
3. To promote settling of vitreous haemorrhage.

A patient presenting with an acute retinal detachment with the macula still attached is operated upon as soon as possible (within 24 hours). While awaiting surgery or if operation has to be delayed for medical or other reasons, then the patient should be immobilised to prevent further extension of the detachment into the macular region. The objective of positioning is to keep the break in the most dependent part of the eye. In the case of a superior break with the risk of rapid extension, the patient must be as flat as possible in the supine position with the head tilted towards the side of the retinal break. Detachments caused by inferior breaks are less likely to be rapidly progressive, but nevertheless the patient should be encouraged to rest quietly in the upright position. Double padding is rarely used.

In a highly myopic patient a superior detachment may be so bullous as to obscure the optic disc and the macula. Bed-rest in the supine position will encourage retina to flatten. This may allow visualisation of the posterior pole, and the exclusion of macular holes or peri-vascular breaks, which may be highly relevant to the planning of surgery. Placing the break in the most dependent position the retina simply falls back as a result of gravity, subretinal fluid flowing relatively easily from subretinal to vitreal compartments particularly through a large retinal break. This process is reversed when the patient resumed an upright position. There is little point in attempting posturing in cases of chronic retinal detachment with small breaks.

On some occasions, by reducing the depth of subretinal fluid, it is possible to convert a case that would otherwise have required drainage of subretinal fluid to aid localisation and to avoid excessive cryotherapy into one where a simple non-drainage procedure may be performed. In patients with acute vitreous haemorrhages and retinal detachment a short period of bed-rest will allow settling of the vitreous haemorrhage to enable a fundal view.

General Medical Treatment

Most cases of retinal detachment require urgent surgery but the need for surgery should not take precedence over essential medical treatment. It may be necessary to defer surgery allowing time for correcting uncontrolled diabetes mellitus, electrolyte imbalance, or the treatment of cardiac arrhythmia and heart failure. Depending on the reason for its use, Warfarin may be stopped for 48 hours prior to surgery. If, however, its continued use is considered advisable then there is no obvious risk of operative haemorrhage if the INR level is kept at 2 to 3. Systemic infections need to be treated. It is unwise to operate on patients with acute upper respiratory tract infections unless it is absolutely necessary. In patients with chronic obstructive airways disease, chest physiotherapy, antibiotics and bronchodilators may improve the pulmonary function prior to surgery. In the medical management of the patient, a co-operative effort of general physicians (calling on the subspecialties particularly of cardiology, respiratory medicine, and diabetology) and of anaesthetists if general anaesthesia is to be used is in the best interest of the patient. It is unusual for these facilities to be available outside a well-staffed general hospital.

Treating Inflammation and Glaucoma

A mild anterior uveitis is often associated with acute retinal detachment and this does not require any specific pre-operative treatment. Reattachment of the retina with surgery usually leads to resolution of the iritis. Chronic retinal detachment can also sometimes present as uveitis. The retinal detachment can escape detection if it is peripherally situated and the fundus not examined with indirect ophthalmoscopy through a dilated pupil.

Occasionally marked inflammatory changes are present (such as combined choroidal and retinal detachment pictures) and these cases are best treated with systemic non-steroidal anti-inflammatory agents combined with intensive topical steroid for a week or more prior to surgery. Mydriatics should be used to dilate the pupil and keep it dilated and hopefully breakdown any posterior synechiae that may have formed.

Secondary glaucoma consequent to inflammatory eye disease or high intraocular pressure associated with severe primary open angle glaucoma should be treated medically with topical therapy or systemic acetazolamide to lower the pressure to near normal levels prior to surgery.

Infection

Periocular infection such as staphylococcal blepharitis or meibomitis is treated to prevent contamination of the surgical field during surgery. Surgery should preferably be delayed and patients are best treated with a topical medication (e.g. chloramphenicol ointment twice daily). At the time of surgery, the lids and the conjunctiva should be cleaned with an antiseptic such as 5% solution of Povidon iodine.

Extruding buckles without obvious sign of infection should be removed prior to surgery, but in the main they do not need to delay surgery, particularly if it is urgently indicated. If there is obvious infection as exemplified by the presence of a mucopurulent discharge from the sinus, a granuloma or the presence of cellulitis, then a preliminary operation should be performed to remove the offending buckle. Definitive intraocular surgery may have to be delayed for 2 weeks to ensure that the wound site is sterile. When removing an infected explant, care should be taken to excise all extra scleral portions of the sutures. If there is infection it is unwise to drag the suture through its scleral track as this may risk intraocular spread.

Obtaining Consent

The informed consent should:

- Be in simple language which a patient can understand
- Include a simple discussion of the diagnosis, the surgery proposed, the likely visual outcome and possible complications
- Confirm the patient's capacity and willingness to receive this information
- Avoid the use of jargon such as 'cryotherapy and plombage', which may mean little to the patient. Abbreviations should be avoided.

It is important to convey possible complications associated with surgery. This should be done in a sensible and sympathetic way, rather than providing the patient with a litany of possible disaster. In general it is reasonable to indicate complications where they have more than a 1% chance of occurring. For example, in the case of vitrectomy performed for the treatment of macular hole, it is reasonable to discuss cataract as a complication but not endophthalmitis.

Similarly when silicone oil is used, it is important to inform the patient of the main complications, e.g. it may be necessary to have a second operation, at the end of say 3–6 months, to remove the silicone oil. Cataract formation occurs in virtually all patients, irrespective of when the oil is removed. When silicone is used as a permanent internal tamponade, then there is an increasing likelihood of developing glaucoma. Most patients require long-term if not life-long follow-up.

When obtaining consent for retinal re-attachment surgery, it is advisable to discuss surgical failure as a possible complication even though the surgeon should convey optimism. Even relatively straight-forward operations, like scleral buckling and non-drainage surgery, may have a failure rate of 5%, effectively, one in twenty cases. Failures occur with more regularity in complex cases, and it is surprising how patients and surgeons are often ill-prepared when this happens. The patient needs to be involved in the decision process of deciding to undergo surgical operation. Patients need to understand that successful treatment depends not only on the skill of the surgeon but on the complexity of the retinal detachment. The patient must countenance the possibility of surgical failure, before signing the consent form and undergoing treatment. It is the responsibility of the surgeon to give a realistic appraisal of the chances of success, and the likely outcome in terms of vision for the eye after surgery.

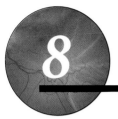

8 Rhegmatogenous Retinal Detachment: Principles of Surgical Management

Principles for Reattachment of the Retina

In RRD, detachment is produced subsequent to break formation. The accumulation of SRF usually results from vitreous traction upon the break and/or the surrounding retina. The treatment of RRD attempts to reverse this process and the principles of treatment involve ways of closing retinal breaks and relieving retinal traction. When RRD is complicated by PVR then surgical reattachment becomes more complex due to the development of additional tractional systems.

Break Closure and Relief of Traction

The aim of surgery is to reattach the retina by means of a series of steps which have the greatest chance of success while incurring the least morbidity. Successful repair of retinal detachment depends on permanent break closure and the relief of traction. Scleral buckling, internal tamponade and vitrectomy combined with retinopexy to achieve sealing of the break are all different means of achieving these objectives. In general the more extensive the surgery the greater the morbidity, thus it is desirable to use the simplest combination of surgical steps.

Relief of Traction Without Break Closure

In repairing retinal detachment uncomplicated by advanced PVR it is desirable but not essential to achieve both objectives of break closure and relief of traction at the time of surgery. Thus, in non-drainage surgery when there is fluid between break and pigment epithelium, the break may still be open at the end of the operation. However, if the buckle is correctly positioned the retinal break will close in the post-operative period, probably due to the relief of vitreo-retinal traction upon it.

Break Closure Without Relief of Traction

An example is pneumatic retinopexy. The tamponade effect of the gas bubble closes the retinal break, but no additional specific measure is used to relieve dynamic traction, although the bubble itself may partially reduce it. When the bubble is absorbed, dynamic traction is reactivated. Although this technique is apparently attractive, the reattachment

> Break closure may be achieved by:
> - Scleral buckles
> - Internal tamponade

rates and complications do not appear to have any advantage over conventional scleral buckling and pneumoretinopexy is not favoured by the authors for the treatment of primary retinal detachment.

Retinopexy

Successful long-term reattachment depends on the formation of a watertight seal of the break through the use of laser photocoagulation or cryotherapy. With either method (laser retinopexy probably acts quicker) secure intraretinal adhesion is not achieved for approximately 2 weeks from the time of application. If, therefore, retinal breaks are not buckled then internal tamponade must be active for this length of time to secure the breaks.

The various methods used to achieve break closure and relief of traction will now be considered in more detail.

The Scleral Buckling Procedure

Modern surgery uses sponge or solid silicone explants to create full-thickness scleral buckling. Questions relating to scleral buckling are (1) how does it cause the relief of dynamic and static traction; and (2) should buckles be applied radially or circumferentially?

Scleral Buckling to Close Breaks and Relieve Dynamic Traction

It is easy to appreciate that scleral buckling resulting in internal indentation may close a retinal break by approximating the pigment layer to the neuro-epithelium. However, it is more difficult to conceptualise how the application of an explant relieves dynamic traction. This pull is strongest, when the vitreous is detached, and exerted acutely at the posterior border of the vitreous base. The vitreous could be pictured as a set of curtains hung on a curtain rail. When the curtain billows in the wind the pull is exerted at the attachment of the curtain, namely the curtain rail. In the eye, the rail corresponds to the vitreous base. When an indent is applied at the vitreous base the highest point of indent is closer to the centre of the globe. The weight of the vitreous is therefore borne by its attachment to the retina adjacent to the indent. If we return to the analogy of the curtain, an indent is pictured as a curtain rail having a downward bend. It is then easy to imagine how the weight of the curtain is taken up by the curtain rail, adjacent to this bend.

Static Traction

When static traction is judged to be present, and has not been relieved by surgical manoeuvres such as epiretinal membrane dissection, permanent buckles are useful to close breaks and to relieve the permanent tractional forces upon them.

Radial vs Circumferential Elements

The vitreous base sits astride the pars plana and the ora serrata over a width of several millimetres. An indent whether it is created by a circumferential or a radial element, would bring the posterior border of the vitreous base closer to the centre of the eye. The weight of the vitreous, and thus the traction upon the retina is transferred to the area of the retina surrounding the indent. With a radial indent, dynamic traction is shifted laterally and anteriorly whereas

> **Circumferential explants are useful when:**
>
> - Two adjacent breaks are separated by less than 2 clock hour (or 8 mm apart on the surface of the sclera)
> - Multiple retinal breaks are in close proximity
> - If a single retina break is situated directly under a rectus muscle

with a long circumferential indent the transfer of traction is only anteriorly.

When treating a retinal tear, the perceived tractional force is acting on the horns of the tear and adjacent retina, therefore greater support may need to be applied anteriorly. For small round holes, anterior support may not be as important.

When a buckle is applied, there is a tendency for the buckle to cause a grove in the sclera along the long axis of the explant. A radially applied element would tend to make a radial groove in the sclera extending anteriorly to the ora serrata, and posteriorly towards the equator. It is, therefore, easier to ensure that the break is supported sufficiently anteriorly when the radial element is used.

In selecting either radial or circumferential buckles the two factors for consideration are: which buckle is best for relieving the traction that is present, and second which buckle is best for achieving break closure considering the various configuration of breaks that may be encountered (Fig. 8.1).

The following is a guide in buckling selection:

- Radial buckles which give good anterior support are useful for single breaks (particularly tears) or two separate tears provided they are separated by a quadrant or so
- Circumferential buckles are indicated when retinal breaks are multiple and in close proximity to each other, or if breaks are closely related to muscle insertions. When adjacent breaks are separated by 2 clock hours (approximately 8 mm apart on the surface of the sclera) or less it becomes awkward to apply multiple radial buckles and circumferential ones should be used.

In some situations the choice between radial and circumferential buckling may not be critical (for example, one or two small round holes in close proximity which can be buckled with either method). Radial buckles tend to produce more astigmatic refractive errors than circumferential ones, but the latter have a greater risk of folding and fish mouthing.

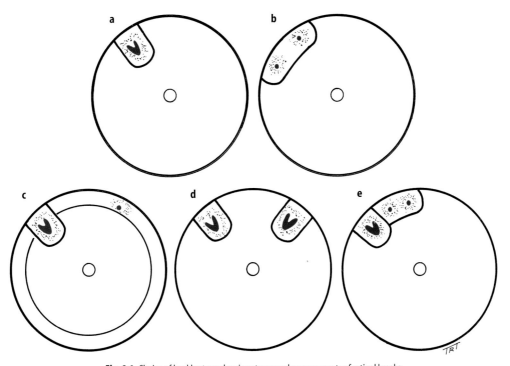

Fig. 8.1. Choice of buckles to seal various types and arrangements of retinal breaks.

Retinal Folds and Fish-Mouthing of Retinal Breaks

This is the formation of retinal folds, which may give rise to the fish-mouthing phenomenon. Scleral buckling greater than 90° effectively shortens the arc of the scleral circumference under the buckle. This shortening tends to give rise to folds in overlying detached retina, running in an axis that is perpendicular to the long axis of the explant (Fig. 8.2). This tendency to folding is accentuated by increasing depth of subretinal fluid. When there is a great depth of subretinal fluid, retinal folds produced by circumferential explants tend to be large and few in number, and when subretinal fluid is shallow, the folds tend to be numerous and occur as small pleats. If retinal breaks are situated on the anterior aspect of the fold, the shape of the break is distorted, giving rise to the appearance of a fish mouth. This tends to prevent break closure and promotes surgical failure. When long circumferential buckles are to be used and subretinal fluid is deep, it is advisable to drain subretinal fluid and perform the D-ACE sequence,

which has as one of its main advantages the avoidance of this complication (see Chap. 10).

Radial explants never extend more than 90° and therefore folds produced by radial elements are insignificant.

Encircling Explants

Encircling explants are part of the historical evolution of retinal detachment surgery. By reducing the circumference of the globe in the plane of the encirclement, the procedure was considered almost mandatory for retinal detachment. However, successful use of local buckles has proved this incorrect and the encirclement procedure is now rarely used for simple cases. If they are employed, silicone rubber bands with underlying rubber tyres are used. The encirclement procedure increases the risk of post-operative complications (See Chap. 11). However, in some cases of RRD without PVR it still does have some use. For example, when multiple breaks are disposed around the twelve o' clock

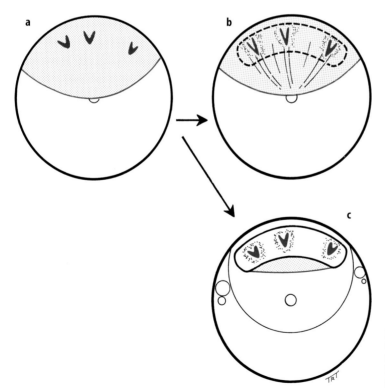

Fig. 8.2. A bullous retinal detachment is present **a**. Circumferential buckling of 90° combined with drainage alone **b** results in multiple radial retinal folds. This will not happen if the D-ACE procedure is used **c**.

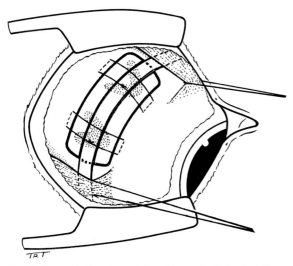

Fig. 8.3. The combination of an encircling rubber band and a localised silicone rubber explant to buckle two adjacent retinal tears.

Indications for encirclement
• To support buckles and tyres in eyes with thin sclera
• For multiple retinal breaks disposed in each quadrant of the fundus
• To support static traction at the vitreous base in anterior PVR

hours it may become impractical to use multiple local buckles. If under these circumstances pars plana vitrectomy is not judged a better method then an encircling tyre of suitable width to give adequate support around each of the tears may be used (Fig. 8.3). This procedure will be combined with drainage of subretinal fluid and air injection into the vitreous cavity as part of the D-ACE procedure. This option is particularly suitable in the very rare cases when sclera is so thin as to be almost impossible to place scleral sutures for the purpose of local buckles.

For eyes with anterior PVR an encircling element is used (usually a 40 or a 240 band) with a wide underlying silicone rubber gutter (e.g. 287) to support the whole area affected by PVR.

Height of Indent

It is necessary to assess the height of the indent required to relieve vitreo-retinal traction and to close a retinal break. The main considerations are the configuration and location of the retinal detachment. The depth of SRF is dependent on the state of the vitreous, thus if the vitreous is very degenerative and collapsed there is a large retrohyaloid space allowing the retina to move forward. Thus the high myope with a degenerate vitreous usually presents with a highly elevated detachment, and a break situated in superior retina, such a break would require a high indent to

achieve break closure, unless SRF was to be drained. This indent would have to be even higher if the break was more posterior and SRF depth even greater.

Inferior retinal breaks seldom produce bullous retinal detachment, even if the vitreous is collapsed. This is because the vitreous gravitates and occupies the lower half of the vitreous cavity reducing the retrohyaloid space and the retinal detachment tends to be shallow. Therefore, inferior retinal breaks require a lower buckle to achieve break closure.

In cases of bullous retinal detachment caused by superior retinal breaks there is a choice between a very high buckle without SRF drainage, or draining SRF and injecting an air bubble. Drainage of SRF and injection of air approximates the break to the underlying pigment epithelium, facilitating and minimising retinopexy. It is then unnecessary to raise anything but a low buckle to maintain break closure, by relieving local vitreoretinal traction .

The following guide is helpful:

- A higher buckle is needed to close a superior break
- A higher buckle is needed to close a posterior break
- A lower buckle will suffice for an inferior and anterior break.

Materials for Buckling

The materials selected for the buckling procedure depend upon the type of case being treated. If SRF is being drained at operation to approximate the break to the pigment epithelium, high buckles are not required and incompressible silicone rubber is perfectly suitable for this purpose. If, on the other hand, it is not possible to close the break at the time of surgery (as in many non-drainage situations) then some expansion of the buckle in the post-operative period is very helpful to achieve break closure. For this, silastic sponge is by far the most suitable material and should be used for most types of non-drainage surgery.

Principles of Internal Tamponade

The object of internal tamponade is to close the retinal break with a bubble of gas or oil until retinoxpexy has sealed the break. Any agent that forms an interface with water may be used for internal tamponade. In practice the choice lies between gaseous agents including air and a variety of inert gases, and silicone fluid. The consequences are:

1. Two immiscible liquids in contact will form an interface
2. Surface tension is generated by attractive forces at the interface (Van de Waal's principle).

Van de Waal's forces are attractive forces between the molecules of the tamponade agent at the interface. These attractive forces act in such a way as to minimise the surface area of the tamponade agent for a given volume, i.e. to form a spherical bubble. When a tamponade agent covers a retinal break, it prevents recruitment of vitreous fluid into the subretinal space through the break. In this way break closure is achieved.

The ability of the tamponade agent to cover the surface of the retina depends on three main factors:

- Contact angles between the tamponade agent and the surface of the retina
- The buoyancy of the agent
- The shape the cavity.

The Contact Angle

When a bubble of tamponade agent is introduced into the eye there is an interaction between three phases in contact with each other. The tamponade effect is determined by the interaction between the retina, the tamponade agent, and its surrounding aqueous. The retinal surface is relatively hydrophilic. Silicone oil being hydrophobic subtends an acute contact angle with the retina. Gases being less hydrophobic make a more obtuse angle with the retina. Therefore for a given volume of internal tamponade agent, gas covers a greater surface of the retina than silicone oil. The contact angles for small bubbles can be predicted by the surface tension alone. For larger bubbles however, other factors become important, and these include the buoyancy, the shape of the vitreous cavity, and therefore the curvature of the retinal surface in contact with the tamponade agent.

Buoyancy

Buoyancy is the difference between the specific gravities of the tamponade agent and the intraocular fluid. The specific gravity of the vitreous fluid in the eye is close to that of water i.e. 1. The specific gravity of air and the various intraocular gases is less than 0.01. Therefore air is very buoyant. A large bubble of air, tends to have a flat lower surface. Where the bubble is very small, (e.g. less than 0.1 ml) then surface energy plays an more important part and the bubble tends to be spherical. Silicone oil has a relatively high specific gravity. (Silicone oils of all viscosity have a specific gravity greater than 0.95). The buoyancy of silicone oil is therefore low and a bubble of silicone oil inside a water-filled cavity such as the eye tends to assume a more spherical shape.

Shape of Cavity

The shape of the vitreous cavity approximates that of a sphere, with the iris-lens diaphragm truncating this sphere and dividing it into an anterior and a posterior chamber. For discussion, the vitreous cavity is assumed to be spherical. The effectiveness of any agent can be described by the relationship between the volume of agent used and the area of retina in contact with the tamponade.

Model eyes constructed of hydrophilic material have been used to study the filling of a spherical cavity with different tamponade agents. The filling characteristics of gas and silicone oil agents are depicted by Fig. 8.4a and Fig. 8.4b, respectively. Fig. 8.4a is a biphasic. The first part of the curve is steep. This explains the fact that a small bubble of tamponade agent can give rise to large area of retinal contact; for example, 0.3 ml covers up to one

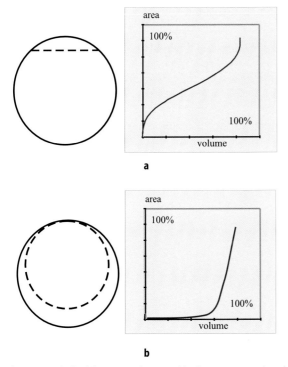

a

b

Fig. 8.4. a A hydrophilic tamponade agent with a large contact angle and high buoyancy (e.g. gas) and consequently the bubble has a virtually bottom surface; **b** shows a hydrophobic tamponade agent (e.g. oil) with a small contact angle and low buoyancy. The bubble has a more spherical shape.

quadrant of the retina. The next part of the curve is virtually linear whilst the last part of the plot rises steeply again. This suggests that a slight under-fill of the cavity would give rise to a disproportionately large area uncovered by a gaseous tamponade agent.

For silicone oil, the filling is represented by Fig. 8.4b. Silicone oil is hydrophobic compared with gas. There is little contact or tamponade effect until the eye is half full. In practice, the aim is to achieve a near complete fill. The right part of the curve is very steep, which again indicates that a slight under-fill would expose a large area not in contact with the oil. The exponential rise of this part of the plot is the consequence of the eye being a near-spherical cavity. Silicone fluid cannot therefore be expected to completely fill the vitreous cavity and eliminate the space into which the retina can detach. Even the best possible clinical fill, inferior breaks (i.e. between the 4 and 8 o'clock hours of the retina) will not be closed and will need to be supported by an additional scleral buckle. Any retinal breaks that are

not covered by the silicone oil will result in recurrent inferior retinal detachment.

Expansion of Gas

Undiluted insoluble gases expand when injected into the vitreous cavity (Fig. 8.5). This expansion is due mainly to the absorption of nitrogen from the blood. The two most popular gases used are sulphahexafluoride (SF6) and perfluoropropane (C3F8). If large volumes of these gases are to be used in the vitreous cavity, then they must be diluted with air so that they remain iso-volumetric, thereby avoiding the risk of subsequent expansion, which may cause glaucoma or central retinal artery occlusion. When the fill is complete, a 20% SF6:air ratio is recommended and a 14% ratio when the gas is C3F8. For PPV uncomplicated by PVR the tamponade only needs to last long enough for the retinopexy to seal retinal breaks. A 20% SF6:air mixture will provide tamponade of superior breaks for approximately 14 days (this time is somewhat shorter in the aphakic eye) . When 14% C3F8 is used the gas remains in the eye for approximately 1 month. Tamponade of breaks below the midline is unreliable for a sufficient length of time for retinopexy to be effective. In these cases additional scleral buckling should be performed.

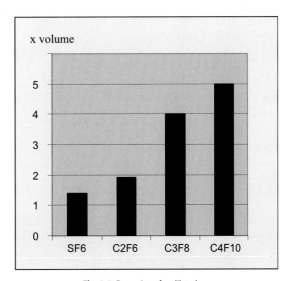

Fig. 8.5. Expansion of undiluted gas.

Principles of Vitrectomy

By carrying out a vitrectomy, the bulk of the vitreous is removed and dynamic vitreo-retinal traction is therefore eliminated. It is then possible to close superior retinal breaks using internal tamponade alone relying on retinopexy to seal the breaks, confident that traction on the breaks cannot be reactivated when the gas bubble absorbs.

Vitrectomy has additional advantages in cases of RRD complicated by PVR. It provides access to the

PPV
• Eliminates dynamic traction
• Allows relief of static traction

retinal surface allowing removal of epiretinal membranes. These are mainly on the pre-retinal surface but they may also be removed from the subretinal aspect of the retina.

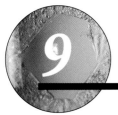

9 Rhegmatogenous Retinal Detachment: Surgical Choices

RRD – Surgical Choices
- Conventional surgery without drainage
- Conventional surgery with drainage
- Pars plana vitrectomy

The pre-operative examination will enable a decision to be made about the type of surgical procedure. This decision will combine the twin objectives of first, using a procedure that carries with it the best chance of surgical reattachment and visual improvement with one operation and second, using the least traumatic and complicated method (Figs. 9.1 and 9.2).

First Decision: Conventional or PPV?

Conventional surgery is suitable for all cases when

- Breaks are not too 'difficult'
- PVR is either absent or poorly developed
- Other unusual features are absent (e.g. intraocular foreign body, IOFB).

PPV is indicated (Fig. 9.3)

1. When breaks are difficult because of:
   - Size (greater than 1 clock hour in diameter)
   - Position (e.g. at the posterior pole)

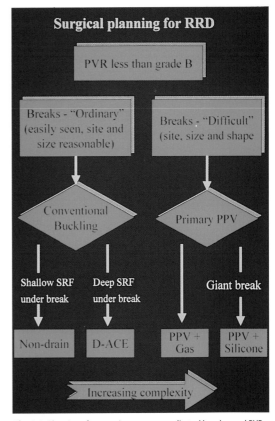

Fig. 9.1. Planning of surgery in cases uncomplicated by advanced PVR.

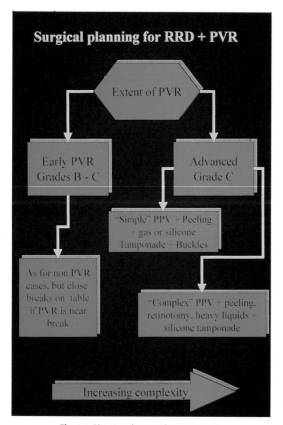

Fig. 9.2. Planning of surgery for RRD and PVR.

- The relationship of breaks to one another (e.g. multiple breaks at different antero-posterior locations)
- Opacities in the media make them unseen or uncertain.

2. PVR: PPV is indicated if PVR is either localised to the posterior pole (macular pucker) or to be sufficiently extensive enough to cause
   - Difficulty in break closure by concealment, distortion or immobilisation of retina near breaks.
   - Sufficient traction upon the retina to prevent retinal reattachment even if break closure can be achieved.

3. The presence of other unusual factors demanding an intraocular approach (e.g. IOFB, extensive choroidal detachment).

Second Decision: Drainage or Non-drainage?

If conventional external surgery is selected the next decision concerns drainage versus non-drainage.
Non drainage is selected if

- SRF between break and pigment epithelium is not deep (Fig. 9.4).
- Break arrangement is not complex
- Retinal mobility in the vicinity of the break is reasonable.

Drainage of SRF (usually combined as part of the D-ACE procedure) is indicated in the following situations:

- Highly elevated breaks (making risk of buckle localisation and retinopexy difficult if non-drainage surgery is attempted)
- The need to close breaks at surgery due to PVR near breaks
- Non-drainage otherwise not indicated (e.g. a rise in intraocular pressure is dangerous)

Decisions 1 and 2 enable a choice to be made between conventional surgery and PPV, and then between the types of conventional surgery. In the majority of ordinary cases these decisions are based on:

- The characteristics of the retinal breaks
- The depth of SRF under the breaks
- The absence or degree of PVR if present

Third Decision: Breaks not seen

When breaks are not seen even after prolonged searching both pre- and per-operatively, and having excluded non-rhegmatogenous detachment the following action is advised (Fig. 9.5):

- Opacities in the media. If these are the cause of the failure to see a break, or if the break that has been seen does not conform to the configuration of the SRF, then in most cases PPV is advised to clear the media and to find the hidden breaks.
- Clear media. If in spite of assiduous searching when the media are clear and there is a good

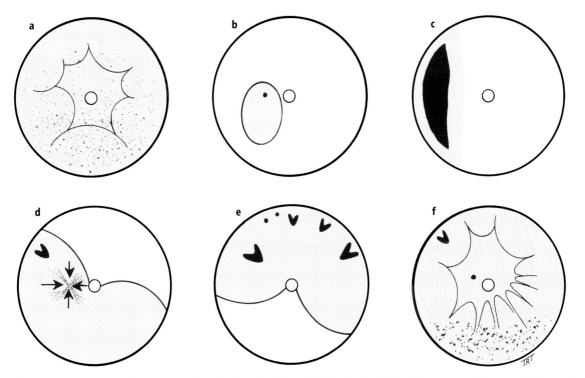

Fig. 9.3. Indications for PPV in RRD: **a** opacities in the media; **b** macular hole causing RRD; **c** giant break; **d** macular pucker; **e** multiple breaks at different levels; **f** RRD complicated by PVR.

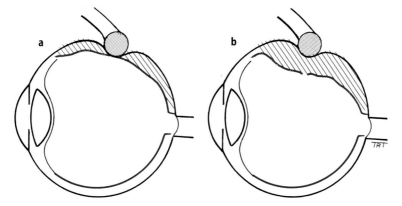

Fig. 9.4. On pre-operative examination the scleral depressor approximates pigment epithelium to the break **a**; non-drainage surgery is indicated. In **b** the intervening SRF is deep and the D-ACE procedure is chosen.

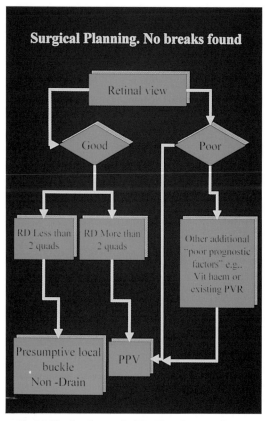

Fig. 9.5. Planning of surgery for RRD without detection of break.

view of detached retina, then breaks must be very small. If RRD is localised (less than two quadrants) then it is reasonable to raise a presumptive buckle (usually a 5-mm pre-equatorial circumferential sponge without drainage of SRF) based on the presumed site of a peripheral break at the posterior border of the vitreous base. If RRD is total or subtotal then presumptive buckling is too speculative and PPV with internal searching is advised. In high myopia (as there is an additional risk of unseen posterior breaks) PPV is more likely to be selected.

10 Rhegmatogenous Retinal Detachment: Conventional Surgery

Conventional surgery consists of external buckling either without drainage of SRF or if SRF is drained with or without added gas injection into the vitreous cavity.

The Non-drainage Operation

Rationale

The accurate placement of a scleral buckle, resulting in closure of the retinal break either at the time of surgery or in the post-operative period will result in spontaneous SRF absorption by the pump action of the pigment epithelium making surgical removal of SRF unnecessary. When SRF is very shallow breaks can easily be closed at the time of surgery but remarkably, even in cases when it is not possible to achieve break closure at the time of operation, a successful outcome will still occur. If the buckle has been placed accurately and is of adequate dimensions the break will gradually sink against the buckle in the post-operative period, and after break closure the remaining SRF will absorb (Fig. 10.1). A little surgical nerve is required!

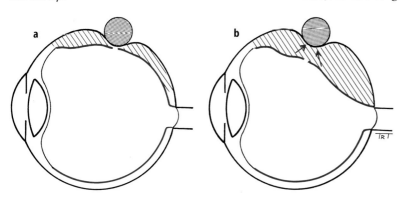

Fig. 10.1. The non-drainage operation. In **a** the break is closed at the time of surgery. In **b** there is intervening SRF but accurate and adequate buckle placement will ensure subsequent break closure.

Advantages

- Drainage of SRF is avoided, and with it related complications (e.g. choroidal haemorrhage, vitreous incarceration, intraocular infection)
- The procedure involves minimal trauma, resulting in a quiet post-operative eye
- In the event of re-operation the surgeon will return to an eye that has not been greatly disturbed by the previous procedure.

Disadvantages

- If SRF between break and pigment epithelium is substantial then accurate localisation of the buckle becomes more difficult

- If it is impossible to close the break at the time of surgery with the cryo-probe then freezing through to the neuro-epithelium will require prolonged application. This rather heavy application may encourage pigment epithelial cells to disperse into the vitreous cavity via the retinal breaks thus tending to promote the process of PVR.
- Buckle height is difficult to estimate and when silastic sponge is being used, it may be higher than expected and may result in significant post-operative astigmatic refractive error.

> Scleral indentation under the break helps gauge SRF depth and indicates feasibility of non-drainage surgery

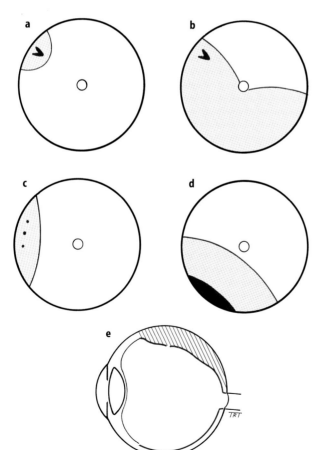

Fig. 10.2a–e. Examples of non-drainage surgery. Local buckles without drainage of SRF can be used, as in all cases depth of SRF under the break is shallow.

Non-Drainage: Yes

The non-drainage retinal detachment operation is suitable for a wide range of simple detachment cases, particularly (Fig. 10.2)

1. When SRF between break and neuro-epithelium is not too deep
2. When the arrangement of the breaks is not too complex
3. When detached retina has not become extensively infiltrated by peri-membranes.

Cases for re-operation and detachments arising in the aphakic or pseudophakic eye are perfectly suitable for non-drainage procedures provided the above criteria are followed.

Non-Drainage: No

1. Difficulty with buckle localisation. Accurate placement of the buckle to seal the retinal break is essential and this accuracy is threatened if
   - Deep SRF intervenes between break and pigment epithelium (Fig. 10.3)
   - Breaks themselves are complex either because of size, or position or arrangement.
2. PVR. Cases with advanced PVR will not be suitable for non-drainage surgery. If breaks are immobilised and distorted by tangential traction or if retina elsewhere is affected, movement of retina towards pigment epithelium is severely impaired. In less advanced cases of PVR (corresponding to approximately C or less of the modern classification), rarely the non-drainage operation may still be used, but only if breaks are not immediately adjacent to peri-retinal

membranes and also if it is judged that the rest of the retina is not irreversibly fixed.

3. Dangers of high intraocular pressure. While buckle sutures are being tightened during a non-drainage operation, intraocular pressure may rise to over 60 mmHg It is dangerous to raise the intraocular pressure to this extent, when there is
   - Unseen optic disc. The disc must be inspected regularly during the non-drainage procedure to check that the central retinal artery is still patent. Operation is precluded if the disc cannot be seen either due to opacities in the media or by overhanging detachment
   - Thin sclera. Tying of the buckle sutures in the non-drainage operation puts considerable tension on the adjacent sclera and if the latter is very thin, it may be impossible to get the sutures to hold.
   - Open angle glaucoma. The outflow channels may be unable to cope with the raised pressure and demand for increased aqueous outflow. The rise of pressure may be therefore unduly prolonged, which not only results in risk of ischaemia of the optic disc, but also in a much longer operating time.
   - Rupture of a recent anterior segment wound. This is not a danger in small incision cataract surgery, but if large wounds are present they may rupture with loss of aqueous and iris prolapse.
   - Ipsilateral poor ocular perfusion. This may result in closure of the central retinal artery as soon as there has been even the slightest rise of intraocular pressure, e.g. in central retinal artery disease or ipsilateral carotid disease. Hypotension during anaesthesia is undesirable and may contribute to marked reduction of perfusion to the eye.

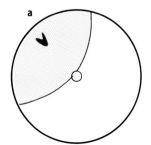 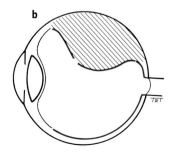

Fig. 10.3. A bullous upper retinal detachment **a**. SRF between break and pigment epithelium is very deep **b**. The D-ACE procedure is indicated.

4. The non drainage operation will rarely be possible in the vitrectomised eye.

Drainage of SRF

The drainage of SRF may usually be part of two different surgical sequences. They are:

1. The drain, air cryo, explant sequence (D-ACE)
2. The cryo, drain buckle sequence.

Per-operative break closure is achieved by air injection into the vitreous cavity and by scleral buckling. This procedure is particularly suitable when there is deep SRF between break and pigment epithelium. The most commonly encountered situation in which the D-ACE sequence is suitable is for bullous upper retinal detachment with superior breaks.

Occasionally, even when SRF between break and pigment epithelium is not particularly deep it is necessary to drain SRF to ensure break closure at operation (due to pre-retinal membrane in close proximity to the break).

Surgical Detail for Conventional Surgery

Anaesthesia

Although local anaesthesia using retro-bulbar, peri-bulbar or sub-Tenon blocks is being used more frequently than a few years ago, general anaesthesia is still the most favoured method and is particularly suitable for long procedures and vitreo-retinal teaching.

Initial Dissection for Conventional Surgery

- Lids: lashes are not cut and a lateral canthotomy only occasionally needed to improve access.
- Cornea: drying is prevented by regular irrigation with balanced salt solution. Sometimes the epithelium will need to be gently scraped off if it becomes cloudy during the course of surgery.

Conjunctival Incision

An incision is made 1–2 mm parallel to the limbus, the incision is extended to just beyond the extraocular muscles guarding the quadrant of sclera to be exposed. A relieving incision is made at each end and extended towards the fornix (Fig. 10.4a). If all quadrants are to be exposed a 360° incision is made with relieving incisions in the 3 and 9 o'clock positions (Fig. 10.4b). The limbal incision allows simultaneous reflection of conjunctiva and Tenon's layer, and at the end of operation these two layers are drawn forward together to provide a thick covering to explants. Sometimes a more posterior incision will be necessary if the limbus is already scarred

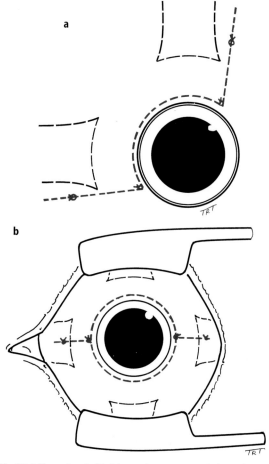

Fig. 10.4. The conjunctival incision used to expose **a** a single quadrant; and **b** all quadrants.

from previous ocular procedures, or if a draining conjunctival bleb from glaucoma surgery is to be avoided.

Isolation of Muscles and Exposure of Sclera

The rectus muscles on either side of where the buckle is to be raised are isolated by blunt dissection and tagged with 3.0 black sutures slipped underneath the muscles on an aneurysm needle. This allows easy rotation of the globe during surgery. During the isolation of muscles stripping all their fascial connections and risking interfering with their blood supply is not necessary.

This dissection is easy in the unoperated eye, but becomes more arduous in those that have undergone previous operations. In these cases, it is often helpful to place a preliminary traction suture at the insertion of the muscle to allow initial rotation of the globe to facilitate access.

Clinical note

- Forceful passage of squint hooks under muscles should be avoided, this move may cause perforation of the globe.
- In re-operations vortex veins may be dragged anteriorly by adhesions from previous operations and may be damaged
- Disinsertion of rectus muscles is never necessary.

Exposure of Sclera

Exposure of sclera is easily achieved in the previously unoperated eye with gentle blunt dissection with a swab after reflection of the conjunctiva and Tenon's layers. Dehiscences or staphylomata with the blue of the choroid showing through thin sclera will be obvious.

Previous Buckling Surgery

If retinal breaks are not situated near the immediate vicinity of old buckles then the latter may be left undisturbed. If on the other hand access to sclera underneath previous buckles is deemed necessary they must be removed with caution. Buckles inserted at previous operations should be approached with care and the following points noted:

- Previous buckles will be found to be surrounded by a reaction tending to enclose the explant in a fibrous tunnel
- They should not be removed at an early stage of the dissection as unexpectedly weak sclera or even choroid may be exposed with the risk of rupture of the globe and loss of SRF or vitreous
- Removal of buckles may result in some degree of hypotony
- Recent sclerotomy sites underneath placed buckles may be re-opened with sudden loss of SRF.

Order of Procedure

After the initial dissection the subsequent order of procedure will depend upon the surgical method that is been chosen.

The Non-drainage Operation

The surgical sequence is:

1. Cryotherapy
2. Break localisation
3. Buckle placement.

Cryotherapy

- Surround the break
- Avoid re-freezing
- Useful for break detection

Cryotherapy

The Break: Indentation with a cryo-probe will approximate pigment epithelium to neuro-epithelium and the break. Thus when freezing occurs it will affect both layers of the retina. The break should be completely surrounded and re-freezing avoided as much as possible. If large breaks are present freezing should be confined to the edges of the break in an attempt to reduce unnecessary disruption of pigment epithelium under the centre of the break. The whiteness of the cryotherapy reaction is due to freezing of the neuro-epithelium. The pigment epithelium itself freezes with a dull grey appearance. For the learning surgeon equatorial breaks are the easiest to treat, as anterior ones (e.g. dialysis) are more difficult to visualise with a consequent tendency to treat posterior to these breaks. In dialyses cryotherapy should be applied to the dialysis edge including the ora serrata at the ends of the break.

Other areas: Cryotherapy may be used to freeze areas of retinal degeneration (e.g. lattice) or areas that are suspicious of harbouring a break. The whiteness of freezing neuro-epithelium contrasts with the dark central area of a breach in continuity of the neuro-epithelium and easily distinguished from small haemorrhages or pigment clumps. However, detection of small breaks can still be very difficult when retina is folded as the freezing reaction may be uneven.

Per-operative Complications of Cryotherapy

These are common to all conventional detachment procedures and are related to either the indentation by the cryo-probe or to the freezing process itself.

Anterior Segment Complications

1. Problems with intraocular lenses
2. Rupture of section

Now that unstable iris clip lenses have been abandoned, dislocation of intraocular lenses is rare. Posterior chamber lenses with an intact posterior capsule are very stable. AC lenses can move on the iris or in the angle and may cause hyphaema. If this does occur viscoelastic material may be injected into the anterior chamber to restore clarity.

Manipulation of the globe during the application of cryopexy may cause rupture of a recent standard size cataract wound with loss of aqueous and iris prolapse. The wound will have to be re-sutured. Small incision cataract surgery has been an important improvement to prevent this complication; a self-sealing wound makes for a stable anterior segment.

Per-Operative Posterior Segment Complications

1. Scleral rupture
2. Haemorrhage: retinal or choroidal
3. Serous choroidal detachment
4. Pigment fallout

Scleral rupture

During the application of cryotherapy the cryoprobe is fused to the wall of the globe by the developing ice ball. At the end of each application this ice ball must be allowed to melt before removing the cryoprobe from the globe and the temptation to crack the probe off the side of the globe must be resisted. Such cracking may result in scleral rupture and choroidal haemorrhage. This is more likely to occur if the underlying sclera is thin.

Haemorrhage

Indentation and freezing underneath a retinal break that has a prominent vessel traversing the break may result in haemorrhage. Although these haemorrhages are alarming, they are rarely severe. Blood will trickle down either the back of the detached posterior hyaloid until it is deposited at the point at which the posterior hyaloid is still attached to retina or may spread into the substance of the gel itself. Firm pressure on the globe is used to discouraged the spread of such haemorrhage.

Choroidal haemorrhage may develop when cryotherapy is applied directly to the vortex veins. Blood passes either into the subretinal space, via the pigment epithelium or remains under the choroid causing a haemorrhagic choroidal detachment. Firm pressure on the globe is again advised to try to reduce the development of these haemorrhages which fortunately are rarely severe.

Serous Choroidal Detachment

This is rare, but may appear a few moments after cryotherapy has been applied and is usually associated with some degree of choroidal haemorrhage. The serous effusion may rapidly become bullous. If the break can be buckled the choroidal detachment will disappear spontaneously in the post-operative period.

Pigment Fallout

Disruption of the pigment epithelium due to cryotherapy may result in pigment granules being exploded into the subretinal space and spreading either via the retinal break into the vitreous cavity or more usually within the subretinal space itself to be deposited at the most posterior part of the retinal detachment. This will often be in the region of the posterior pole in the supine patient. Pigment fallout is produced either as a result of excessive or repeated applications of cryotherapy, or due to perfectly normal applications in eyes where the pigment epithelium appears to be unusually loose (e.g. as in longstanding retinal detachments). In these cases pigment epithelium can actually be seen entering the vitreous cavity via the retinal break shortly after the cryo-probe has been applied. Pigment fallout does not appear to jeopardise post-operative visual acuity even if it occurs in the para-macular region. Pigment released into the subretinal space is often seen flowing out if SRF is drained after cryotherapy.

Technique of Break Localisation

In previously unoperated eyes retinal breaks are localised under indirect ophthalmoscopic observation using a modified scleral depressor, which when indented vertically on to the sclera leaves a small circular impression (Fig. 10.5). The centre of this impression is then marked with a methylene blue pencil leaving an identifiable spot on the sclera. In re-operations when the scleral surface is uneven or when the eye is soft and the sclera not easily marked by the depressor, localisation may be achieved by grasping the sclera with toothed forceps, the position of which may be changed until accurately sited.

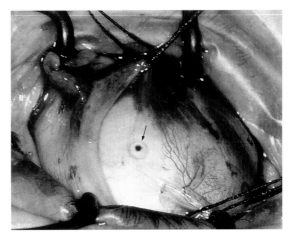

Fig. 10.5. Break localisation.

When breaks are small a single mark is all that is needed, made just under the break. The mark will be the central point of the mattress suture being used to raise the buckle. However, if the break is large, multiple markings may be necessary. Thus with large retinal tears, one mark may be at the posterior part of the break and the other two placed at the anterior extremities. In dialysis, two anterior marks are made at each end and one in the mid-point of the posterior edge of the dialyses.

Accurate localisation of retinal breaks requires expert indirect ophthalmoscopy and emphasises the need for development of these skills by assiduous pre-operative examination.

Scleral Buckling in Non-drainage Surgery

- Sutures
- Selection of explants
- Handling of the explant
- Raising of the buckle
- Raise of intraocular pressure
- Accidental perforation.

Sutures

The most satisfactory sutures for securing local sponge explants are 5/0 braided Dacron on a spatulated needle (either a quarter or half-circle). The quarter circle needle is preferred when there is good scleral access allowing long scleral bite. The half circle needle is particularly valuable when access to the dissection site is difficult (e.g. near a muscle or in a posterior position).

Technique (Fig. 10.6)

When placing the sutures the intrascleral course should be as long as possible (approximately 5 mm), thereby reducing the risk of sutures cutting out either when they are tightened at the time of surgery or in the post-operative period, to contribute to explant extrusion. When placing the suture the sclera is made firm and stationary by counter

traction by non-toothed forceps on an adjacent rectus muscle insertion. Counter traction will also straighten the sclera so that the normal curvature of the globe is less pronounced, making for easier passage of the needle. In sclera of normal thickness the suture runs at approximately two-thirds of the scleral thickness. At this depth the suture will be just detected in its intrascleral course. The placement of these sutures is a matter of fine judgement: too deep a suture will cause accidental perforation with subsequent release of SRF, while too shallow a suture will cut out. Sutures are arranged in mattress fashion to straddle the intended explant and are held provisionally in bulldog clips until tied permanently (these may be colour coded for rapid identification).

Width of Suture

A general rule is to place the sutures approximately half as wide again as the width of the explant, (thus for a 4-mm explant the limbs of the sutures 6 mm apart, for a 5-mm explant 8 mm apart and for a 7-mm explant 10 mm apart). The break should lie in the centre of the buckle.

Complications

Vortex veins may be damaged in the following ways:

- Their intrascleral course may be damaged as the needle passes through the sclera
- Damage may occur as the needle is removed from the sclera in their vicinity
- The vortex veins, adherent to the loose periocular fascia, may be dragged into the suture track by the trailing thread as the suture is pulled from the sclera.

If the needle is nearing a tributary of the vortex vein it is removed from the sclera, passed over the vein, and reintroduced into the sclera on the other side of the vein. If a vortex vein is damaged during dissection resulting in bleeding, it is better to leave it to cease spontaneously rather than try to stop the flow of blood by compression or diathermy which may risk intraocular haemorrhage.

Accidental perforation: In an intended nondrainage operation, accidental perforation of the globe with release of SRF is always disappointing.

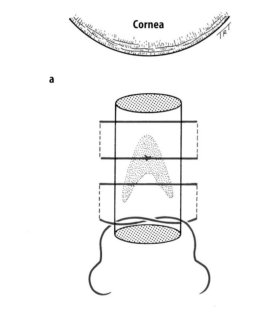

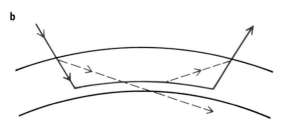

Fig. 10.6. a Technique for sutures for radial buckling. **b** Correct suture plane is shown by the continuous line. The dotted line runs the risk of sutures cutting out or, if too deep, of perforating the eye.

However, due to the small puncture site, incarceration of the retina and vitreous loss will not occur, unless perforation has occurred over flat retina. If accidental perforation of the subretinal space occurs the suture should be removed and the leak of SRF sealed by oversewing with a more widely placed suture. However, if previous pressure inside the eye has been elevated by the tightening of previous sutures release of SRF may be rapid and the eye will rapidly become hypotonic. In these cases intraocular pressure should be restored by the intra-vitreal injection of air converting the operation into a modified form of the D-ACE procedure.

Selection of Explants

In non-drainage surgery silastic sponge explants are usually preferred (Fig. 10.7a). The elastic nature of this material allows for some post-operative expansion of the buckle, a feature that is important when it is not possible to close the break completely at the

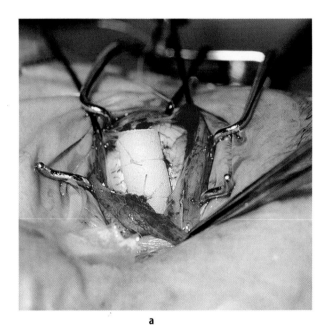

a

Fig. 10.7. a Radial sponge buckling. **b** A circumferential sponge used to close a dialysis in (i) and is also useful in closing several round holes in (ii).

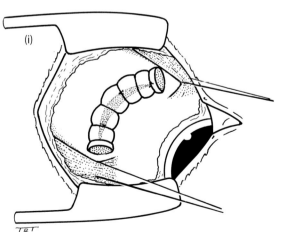

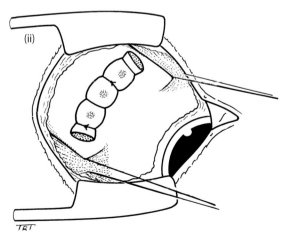

b

Accidental drainage of SRF
● Remove suture and oversew
● Inject air into vitreous if the eye becomes soft

time of surgery. However, if break closure is easy at the time of surgery, and only a low buckle is required, then solid silicone rubber explants may be used. It is extremely unusual for an encirclement procedure to be necessary as part of a non-drainage operation.

Size of Explant

The buckle selected must not only be accurately placed, but must be of sufficient dimensions to seal the retinal breaks. Explants of 4 mm and 5 mm widths are by far the most commonly used, but for larger breaks the 7-mm sponge explant may be necessary. The selection of the size of buckles should result in a buckle of adequate but not excessive proportions (Fig. 10.7b).

Handling the Explant

To reduce the risk of contamination the sponge should not be removed from its sterile package until just before its introduction to the eye. Prior to its placement on the eye it is soaked in a broad spectrum antibiotic (e.g. cefuroxime) and during manipulation it is held in non-toothed forceps to avoid damage and disruption of its cellular structure.

Raising of the Buckle

For radial buckles the posterior suture is tightened first (this is where most indentation is needed) and for circumferential buckling the middle suture is tied first if three are needed. As sutures are tied there is a tendency for poorly secured ones to cut out. The tying of the first suture is achieved without difficulty in an eye that is fairly soft but subsequent sutures are more difficult as the intraocular pressure rises. These are best secured with temporary knots (a single tucked reef) which can easily be released if

intraocular pressure is high, preventing arterial perfusion of the disc.

Rise of Intraocular Pressure

With successive tightening of the sutures the intraocular pressure rises and this may cause central retinal artery occlusion. Of lesser importance is corneal oedema which will contribute to diminution of the fundal view. Intravenous diamox 500 mg given at the beginning of surgery helps lower intraocular pressure.

If general anaesthesia is to be used, hypotension is undesirable, as it may lead to reduced perfusion of the optic disc.

Action:

● Massage of the globe with a squint hook increases aqueous output and lowers intraocular pressure. If central retinal artery occlusion has occurred spontaneous pulsation of the artery may be observed after a few seconds of massage
● If massage does not produce perfusion, then temporary suture is released
● Paracentesis. If the buckling procedure is to be unusually extensive and disc perfusion is uncertain then paracentesis may be performed in the phakic or pseudophakic eye. It should be avoided in the aphakic eye as vitreous may be incarcerated into the limbal incision
● Corneal oedema resulting from intermittent rise of intraocular pressure may necessitate removal of the corneal epithelium.

Problems with Buckle Placement

1. Inadequate buckle
2. Radial retinal folds.

Inadequate Buckle

A buckle may be classed as inadequate if it is inaccurately placed or is of insufficient dimensions to close the retinal breaks. Satisfactory buckling will usually be obvious if it is possible to close breaks at the time of surgery. However, with non-drainage procedures when there is still intervening SRF between buckle and neuro-epithelium inaccurate buckling is more likely.

Radial Retinal Folds

As discussed in Chap. 8, circumferential buckling of approximately one segment of sclera may result in radial retinal folds, a tendency that is more pronounced when there is deep SRF. Small folds are of no clinical importance and will flatten out spontaneously in the post-operative period as SRF is absorbed. If prominent they may allow communication between the posterior part of a break and SRF behind the buckle. Radial buckling will not result in radial folds but if this option is not reasonable then the D-ACE sequence should be performed.

The D-ACE Sequence

This sequence consists of:

- Drainage of SRF
- Air injection into the vitreous cavity
- Cryotherapy
- Explant.

Rationale

The rationale of this sequence is that drainage of SRF will create space within the eye to enable an injection of air into the vitreous cavity. The bubble of air pushes the detached retina back towards the pigment epithelium. Once the retinal break is in contact with pigment epithelium or very nearly so cryotherapy can be applied and a buckle used to keep the break sealed by relieving traction upon it. In this sequence, the air injection is used mainly as a per-operative tool and, in view of the fact that it is absorbed quite quickly in the post-operative period, it is doubtful that it has anything more than a temporary post-operative tamponade effect.

Site for Drainage of SRF

Prior to drainage the site to be chosen should be under deep SRF in the equatorial or pre-equatorial region. If the drainage site is too anterior then the flow of SRF may cease due to closure of the sclerotomy by the enlarging air bubble after injection into the vitreous cavity as it is anterior retina that is first compressed by the bubble. Drainage of fluid under a large retinal break should be avoided for fear of incarceration of the posterior hyaloid through the retinal break into the sclerotomy. For superior bullous detachments drainage above the midline will be the rule, and if possible the upper temporal quadrant should be selected. Access is easier in this quadrant and there is less risk of haemorrhage than in the nasal quadrant where vortex veins are more numerous.

SRF drainage site
● Under deep SRF
● Avoid vortex veins
● Avoid large breaks
● Post-equatorial

The authors currently favour two methods of drainage of SRF and air injection, described below.

Method 1

A radial incision in the sclera is made at the selected site with a size 11 Bard Parker blade. The incision should be long enough to expose a reasonable knuckle of choroid. A 5.0 Dacron suture on a half-circle needle is then placed across the lips of the wound. This stitch is of considerable importance; if insecurely tied raising of intraocular pressure when the eye is buckled after air injection may result in prolapse of vitreous and retina through the sclerotomy.

Transillumination

With the operating theatre darkened the sclerotomy is then transilluminated by shining a fibre-optic light through the pupil via the cornea. Large choroidal vessels crossing the exposed choroidal knuckle can be clearly seen (Fig. 10.8). If these are numerous and are likely to be damaged by

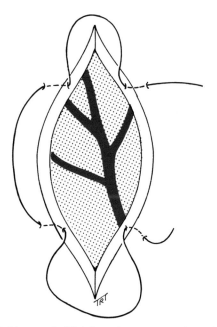

Fig. 10.8. Sclerotomy for SRF drainage. A mattress suture is pre-placed. A large vein is seen in the choroid.

perforation of the choroid or if during the preparation of the drainage site there has been spontaneous external bleeding then the wound should be secured and a further site selected.

Perforation of Choroid

If no blood vessels can be seen, the knuckle is cauterised to discourage bleeding. The subretinal space will often be entered during the process of cautery, but if it is not, the final perforation may be achieved by sharp needle puncture.

Character of SRF

In fresh retinal detachment the SRF will have a watery consistency, but in longer standing cases the fluid will be viscous and xanthochromic.

Complications of SRF Drainage

- Choroidal haemorrhage
- Retinal haemorrhage
- Cessation of flow
- Retinal incarceration.

Choroidal Haemorrhage

Choroidal haemorrhage is the most important and dangerous complication of SRF drainage (Fig. 10.9). It may occur either at the time of perforation of the choroid and release of SRF, in which case it is related to direct damage to a choroidal blood vessel or during SRF drainage when hypotony is probably a contributory factor. If blood is seen to be emerging in the SRF then it is likely that there will have been intraocular spread. Choroidal bleeding will usually pass into the subretinal space and track downwards to the most dependent part of the globe. Sometimes it passes through the retinal break into the vitreous cavity. If the macula is detached blood will tend to settle in the macular region and threaten subsequent recovery of central visual acuity. Rarely haemorrhagic choroidal detachment may occur and be seen as a black mound beneath the detached retina.

In most cases haemorrhage although alarming, will be slight and will not interfere with break closure or increase the risk of redetachment.

Action: If haemorrhage starts as soon as the subretinal space is entered, then firm pressure on the side of the eye will encourage egress of blood from the eye in the SRF and will prevent the eye from becoming too soft. Air injection should be carried out as soon as possible. In the rare event of blood

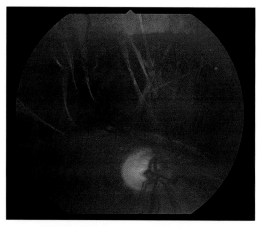

Fig. 10.9. Haemorrhage in the subretinal space.

spreading into the vitreous cavity and interfering with the view, the D-ACE operation may have to be abandoned in favour of a pars plana vitrectomy.

Retinal Haemorrhage

Rarely severe haemorrhage may result from direct trauma by the perforating needle to the underlying retinal blood vessels. Such trauma usually leads to the formation of jagged iatrogenic breaks and severe vitreous haemorrhage.

> Intraocular haemorrhage is the most serious complication of SRF drainage

Cessation of Flow

Flow of SRF may cease abruptly and if so the intraocular situation should be checked. If SRF drainage is considered sufficient the drainage site can be closed. If SRF drainage is deemed inadequate, the flow of SRF may be recommenced by gently manipulating the lips of the sclerotomy or by re-perforation with a needle. It is essential to check that there is still reasonable depth of SRF between the sclerotomy site (seen as a white mark when viewed with the indirect ophthalmoscope) and the detached retina before this move is made.

Retinal Incarceration

This is easily recognised as the retina has a thin greyish appearance at the sclerotomy site when viewed externally and on indirect ophthalmoscopy (Fig. 10.10) the typical puckering into the sclerotomy site is seen. This appearance is further accentuated by vitreous incarceration and loss, which frequently accompanies retinal incarceration. Retinal incarceration is due to poor surgical technique and may occur in a variety of ways:

- Improper selection of drainage site
- Raised intraocular pressure.

Improper selection of drainage site: If the retina is flat at the site that has been chosen for drainage of

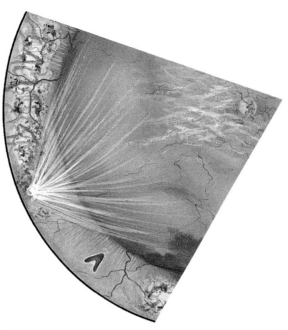

Fig. 10.10. Incarceration of retina and vitreous has occurred at an SRF drainage site.

SRF, perforation of the choroid will be succeeded by that of the retina, with a resulting loss of vitreous through the sclerotomy. If SRF is very shallow at the site of drainage, retina may be incarcerated after the flow of SRF has started.

Raised intraocular pressure: The drainage site is left open during air injection and over-injection may force retina into the sclerotomy.

Action: No attempt should be made to free the retinal incarceration from the sclerotomy site which should be supported by a buckle to counteract secondary traction at the site of incarceration and to close any iatrogenic break that occurs if vitreous is lost. It is unnecessary to apply cryotherapy unless an iatrogenic break is seen.

Intravitreal Injection of Air

- Preparation
- Injection site
- Technique for injection.

Preparation

The air is drawn up into a sterile freely running dry glass syringe through a 0.22 Millipore filter. The syringe is tested by the surgeon prior to use to gauge the force necessary in the plunger to start the injection. A syringe that tends to stick and cause hesitant injection of gas is to be avoided. A 27-gauge needle is used.

Injection Site(Fig. 10.11)

The needle needs to be uppermost at the time of injection and this is most easily achieved by injecting through the superior pars plana while the eye is turned down. The upper nasal quadrant is the most convenient and the needle is introduced 4 mm from the limbus.

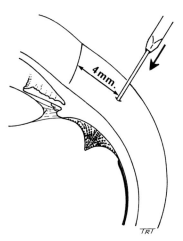

Fig. 10.11. Injection of air via the pars plana. The needle must perforate the non-pigmented part of the pars plana epithelium.

Technique of Injection

This is performed under indirect ophthalmoscopic control. In spite of gentle pressure on the eye during the evacuation of SRF, this pressure will have to be released just prior to the injection of air and at this moment the globe will be very soft. The insertion of an adjacent rectus muscle should be grasped to allow counter traction and to enable downward rotation of the eye prior to the introduction of the 27-gauge needle into the vitreous cavity. A sharp thrust ensures that the needle tip has entered the vitreous cavity and is not tenting up the non-pigmented part of the pars plana epithelium. The direction of the needle is towards the centre of the vitreous body to avoid damage to the lens. As soon as the tip of the needle is seen further rotation of the eye may be achieved so that the syringe comes to occupy as vertical a position as possible. The needle is then withdrawn so that only the tip is visible and the injection commenced at a steady speed. If the needle is correctly positioned than an intravitreal gas bubble can be seen forming in the immediate vicinity of the needle tip and progressive injection will then produce a single gas bubble, in to which the needle tip can be advanced as the injection proceeds. With this technique multiple bubbles are avoided (Fig. 10.12).

Volume to be Injected

Intraocular pressure is monitored with a fingertip during injection. Air injection should cease when the eye is considered to be just hypotensive. The volume of air that will be necessary to achieve this will vary greatly from one case to another, usually

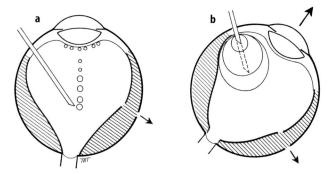

Fig. 10.12. Injection of air. **a** Incorrect technique results in multiple bubbles in the vitreous cavity; **b** correct technique with the needle in the "high" position and the eye rotated. The needle tip is advanced into the enlarging air bubble and results in a single intraocular bubble.

1–2 ml are needed. Fundoscopy will reveal whether the objective of the air injection (to approximate the retinal break to the underlying pigment epithelium) has been achieved. If this is so, then the drainage site should be closed and no further air injection will be necessary. However, if there is still substantial SRF between break and pigment epithelium then more SRF is drained and further air injection is carried out until break closure occurs.

Difficulties

Drainage of SRF followed by air injection requires organisation and good technique and this is the most difficult part of the operation to master. After the injection of air there will be minification of retinal landmarks including retinal breaks and these breaks may be difficult to find. Sometimes after SRF drainage and air injection the volume of SRF will be unchanged. This is due to retro-hyaloid fluid draining directly through the sclerotomy via a big retinal break; if this happens, allow more SRF drainage and top up the air injection.

Air injection technique
● Check syringe and needle
● Upper nasal quadrant is preferred
● Needle as vertical as possible
● Direct needle away from lens
● Monitor intraocular pressure during injection
● Stop injection when break has reached pigment epithelium

Method 2

Technique for Drainage

Drainage of SRF is achieved by means of a 27-gauge needle. The site of drainage should be over an area of deepest SRF. The needle is pre-bent at a right-angle 2 mm from the tip. The needle is used to penetrate the full thickness of the sclera in one firm continuous action. The needle is held in place momentarily and withdrawn. Digital pressure is immediately applied to the globe and sustained for a full 5 minutes. At the end of 5 minutes the pressure is released. If intraocular haemorrhage is observed then digital pressure is resumed for another 2 minutes. Observation is made with an indirect ophthalmoscope. The aim is to achieve not only closure of the central retinal artery but complete blanching of the choroid. Drainage of SRF is followed by injection of air to restore intraocular volume and pressure. This technique has a number of advantages:

● Low incidence of intraocular haemorrhage. This is a result of the sustained intraocular pressure

● Low risk of vitreo-retinal incarceration due to the fact that the perforation of the choroid is a micro-puncture

● Low incidence of retinal perforation due to the fact the needle only penetrates to a preset depth of 2 mm

● Can be safely performed before or after cryotherapy.

The technique relies on two basic premises. First, bleeding cannot occur when the intraocular pressure exceeds that of choroidal arterial pressure. Second, if this pressure is sustained beyond that of the choroidal bleeding time then bleeding should not occur when the digital compression is released. The incidence of bleeding is rare after 5 minutes of digital pressure.

No scleral cut down is necessary. The small puncture by the needle means that vitreo-retinal incarceration is virtually impossible. The pre-bent needle tip prevents deep penetration of the needle and retinal perforation. The drainage of SRF is usually complete.

Dry Tap

On the rare occasion of a dry tap, this is usually because the needle tip has not penetrated the full thickness of the sclera and choroid. Indirect ophthalmoscopy should be performed again to locate the site of deepest SRF. It is important, however, to keep up the digital pressure in between attempts at drainage.

Air Injection

Air injection is accomplished by means of a continuous air infusion pump. To obtain a simple bubble, it is necessary to:

- Adopt the 'needle high position'
- Inject at speed.

The speed of the air injection is determined by the differential pressure. The air pump is set at 60 mmHg but it is also important to lower the intraocular pressure suddenly by releasing the digital compression suddenly.

Complications of Air Injection

Multiple Bubbles

The occurrence of multiple bubbles is as a result of incorrect position of the needle prior to injection and therefore represents poor surgical technique. This complication is particularly worrying if it is obscures details of the underlying retina.

Action: Continue to drain SRF until the eye gets softer and then inject again making sure that the needle position is correct. This second injection should produce one large central bubble and even if there are one or two residual satellite bubbles the view of the underlying retina will usually be adequate enough to enable cryotherapy and explant placement. Rarely small bubbles of air may get through a large retinal break to gain the subretinal space.

Over-injection

Over-injection with a consequent rise of intraocular pressure may cause:

- Retinal incarceration through an unclosed sclerotomy site
- Cession of flow in the central retinal artery
- Forward movement of the lens iris diaphragm may occur and while this is usually unimportant may cause dislocation of unstable pseudophakic lenses, (a haptic may move forwards of the iris) or may result in pupil capture.

It should be remembered that if air is injected into the eye and nitrous oxide is being used as part of general anaesthesia the gas will tend to pass into the air bubble during surgery enlarging it and making the eye firmer.

Action: Passive partial evacuation of a gas bubble may be performed using a needle. Release of a finger placed over the hub will result in escape when the needle has been placed within the intravitreal bubble.

Air Entering the Anterior Chamber

The D-ACE procedure should not be used in the aphakic eye for fear of air passing into the anterior chamber and completely obscuring the view.

Haemorrhage

Haemorrhage from the injection site may occur but is usually slight.

Needle Problems

Poor technique may result in air being injected under the choroid or the non-pigment epithelium and damage to the lens or retina may be caused by a poorly directed needle tip.

Cryotherapy

After drainage of SRF and injection of air, cryotherapy is applied to the retinal breaks that are now apposed to the pigment epithelium. In addition to complications previously described the minified view of the retina may cause difficulty in break detection. The freezing reaction in the retina is intensified as air is a poor heat conductor and this risks excessive freezing. Cryotherapy should also be applied to breaks or areas of lattice degeneration in detached or flat retina.

Explant

A feature of the D-ACE procedure is that subsequent to the approximation of the retinal breaks to the pigment epithelium, it is not necessary to raise high buckles. Thus solid silicone explants are the most suitable, and although various sizes are available the 287 (width of 7 mm) will suit most cases. These buckles are secured using half-circle Dacron sutures. The scleral length of the suture can be quite short (1–2 mm) and as the explant is 7 mm wide the limbs of the suture should be 10 mm apart. Complications of suture placement have already been described, but damage to vortex veins is particularly likely to occur with the posterior limb of the suture if a wide explant is used.

The Encircling Procedure

The success of the simple external local buckles and the use of PPV for complex break arrangement has reduced the need for encircling buckles. If used they should be combined with local buckles, the encirclement only being used to retain the local buckling element. The occasional retinal surgeon will use the encirclement in the mainly mistaken belief that it will serve to close breaks that have not been detected. In these circumstances the encirclement will be usually be excessively tightened, risking severe complications. Used correctly the encircling element (usually a 2-mm silicone band) tied in a quadrant other than the one in which the underlying local explant is being used, will result in an indentation 1–2 mm in height (after tightening, ophthalmoscopy should reveal only a very low indent).

In the D-ACE sequence the encircling band fits into the groove of a solid silicone explant orientated circumferentially. If the explant is confined to one quadrant, the two mattress sutures retaining it should be tied first, before the silicone band is tightened. The band is then lightly secured in each of the three remaining quadrants by small mattress sutures (these sutures should be 12 mm from the limbus). The ends of the strap are cinched together with a silicone rubber sleeve. This allows for adjustment in the tension of the band before it is finally secured.

Variation In the D-ACE Sequence

Longer Acting Gases (e.g. SF6)

The use of a gas longer acting than air may occasionally be helpful if difficulty with break closure is anticipated due to the presence of pre-retinal membrane in the vicinity of the break. In these situations a 30% air:SF6 mixture may be used, this will enable post-operative tamponade of the break to be performed for a period of approximately 1 week from surgery.

The Cryotherapy, Drain, Buckle Sequence

This sequence is reserved for those infrequent cases of retinal detachment where it is deemed necessary to drain SRF (e.g. the presence of membranes in close proximity to breaks) and in which the release of SRF is judged to be too small to create enough space to enable injection of air into the vitreous cavity.

Cryotherapy

Cryotherapy is applied to the retinal breaks prior to the drainage of SRF.

Sutures

The buckle sutures are pre-placed and the buckles themselves (either encircling or local, or both) are placed in position.

Drainage of Fluid

SRF is now drained at a convenient point.

The D-ACE sequence

- The SRF drainage site must be carefully selected
- A single-bubble injection technique must be acquired
- Breaks are minified by the intravitreal air bubble
- Cryo-reaction is intensified
- Only low buckles are required

Tightening of Sutures

As SRF drains from the eye the buckle sutures are tightened. SRF drainage in these cases will not usually be copious and the hypotony induced by SRF drainage is equalised by the tying of the buckle sutures. An injection of air or an air:SF6 mixture is performed if hypotony is greater than anticipated.

Results

Anatomical success with one operation should be achieved in about 90% of cases.

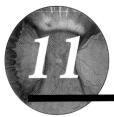

11 Conventional RRD Surgery: Post-operative Management, Signs and Complications

General Aspects of Post-Operative Care

General aspects of post-operative care involve mobilisation, posture, medication and consideration of post-operative activity. If surgery is successful, recovery of vision will commence immediately.

Mobilisation

If general anaesthesia has been used patients are mobilised on the same or the day following surgery, to minimise the risk of thrombo-embolism in the legs. There is no place for post-operative bed-rest and the belief that bed-rest may encourage residual SRF absorption is mistaken. Discharge from hospital depends less on an ophthalmic need than on social convenience and the availability of any necessary help at home.

Posture

Posturing is unnecessary in non-drainage surgery and has a doubtful part to play when air is injected into the vitreous cavity. The gas bubble is rapidly absorbed and the success of the D-ACE procedure depends on accurate localisation of the scleral buckle rather than any contribution made by the bubble.

Medication

A steroid antibiotic drop administered four times a day is suitable for dealing with the variable amount of post-operative external inflammation that is present. Inadvertent freezing of the lids by poor insulation of the cryo probe may cause marked post-operative lid oedema and in severe cases burns to the lid margins. These changes are not permanent, but lead to discomfort in the post-operative period. The external signs are related to the type of procedure that is being performed a more wide spread disturbance being produced with extensive buckling procedure and in re-operations. Conjunctival chemosis is worse following re-operations. Mydriasis is helpful for a few days in all cases (cyclopentolate 1% twice a day is suitable and atropine 1% can be used in more inflamed eyes). Immediate post-operative pain is usually well controlled by the administration of Voltarol administered as a suppository at the end of the surgical procedure. Systemic medication usually consists only of analgesic tablets for a few days, but occasionally post-operative pain will demand analgesia for days or weeks following surgery. In these cases, particularly when inflammation is present, the administration of systemic non-steroidal anti-inflammatory drugs (e.g. Froben 25 mg tds or Indomethacin 50 mg tds). will be helpful.

Post-Operative Activity

Reading may be resumed as soon as it is comfortable so to do. Physical activity can be allowed immediately, but patients will not usually wish to indulge in strenuous activity in the immediate post-operative period. Activity such as heavy lifting, riding or strenuous ball games is not advised for the first few weeks. The length of time that a patient has to remain off work will depend to extent on the type of job and the nature of the operation performed. In uncomplicated cases work may resume approximately 1–2 weeks after surgery, but this interval may have to be lengthened if special visual tasks are to be performed. The patient may later return to all activities of their choice, although sports in which direct damage to the eye is a reasonable possibility should be allowed only if protective eye wear is available. Women of childbearing age should be informed that retinal detachment surgery in no way influences the management of labour of a subsequent pregnancy.

Recovery of Vision

Field of Vision

Restoration of field of vision conforming to the area of retinal detachment occurs almost immediately after successful surgery. Occasionally a faint shadow in the field of vision corresponding to the area of retinal detachment may persist for a few days or weeks following retinal reattachment.

Central Vision

If the macula is detached prior to surgery, the recovery of central visual acuity subsequent to reattachment is variable. The most important factor in determining visual recovery is the length of time that the macula has been detached prior to surgery, the longer detached the poorer the eventual recovery. Recovery is also less satisfactory in old age and myopia. If the macula has been detached for less than 2 weeks then 80% of patients may be expected to achieve a visual acuity of 6/18 or better following reattachment. Although the majority of the restoration of visual acuity takes place within 3 months, the final recovery may be slow and may take up to 2 years from the time of surgery. Improvement in colour discrimination likewise occurs over a long period of time.

Post-Operative Visual Symptoms

- Persistence of pre-operative symptoms
- New symptoms
- Reduction of vision

Persistence of Pre-Operative Symptoms

If a patient had experienced flashes of light with the onset of a posterior vitreous detachment these flashes usually, but not always, disappear with the onset of the retinal detachment and they may reappear in the post-operative period. These symptoms, although alarming, do not usually persist and pass off within few weeks of surgery. Vitreous floaters will not usually be affected by a conventional operative procedure and patients should be warned that they will persist. Indeed, on some occasions they worsen (particularly if pigment is dislodged by cryotherapy and enters the vitreous via the retinal breaks). These floaters tend to improve in the weeks and months following surgery, but may not altogether disappear.

New Symptoms

In cases where retinal detachment has not been associated with the premonitory symptoms of flashes and floaters either or both of these may appear in the post-operative period even when there has been successful and permanent reattachment of the retina. These symptoms tend to ameliorate in the weeks following surgery.

Reduction of Vision

Patients with peripheral retinal detachment and normal acuity prior to surgery may report reduced central vision after operation. Unless a problem has arisen at the macula this reduction is associated with a refractive error induced by the buckling procedure. This error needs correcting by adjusting the spectacle prescription at a later date, but patients should be warned pre-operatively of the likelihood of this event.

Intraocular Signs

- The cryotherapy lesion
- Behaviour of SRF
- PVR

The Cryotherapy Lesion

In successful cases the break will be sited accurately on the buckle and sealed. The pigmentation of the cryo-lesion appears at the end of the first week and has a pepper and salt appearance, which gradually gives way to a coarser arrangement of pigment after a period of weeks. Heavy cryotherapy application causes a production of a very pale lesion due to the destruction of chorio-capillaries and thinning of neuro-epithelium. The maximum strength of the cryotherapy lesion takes approximately 2 weeks to develop.

Behaviour of SRF

The post-operative absorption of SRF following either a non-drainage operation or residual SRF following a drainage procedure depends mainly upon the relationship of the break to the buckle at the end of surgery. If break closure has been achieved at the time of surgery, then SRF absorption will be rapid, and is usually complete within a few days of surgery. Absorption of SRF is delayed if pigment epithelium function is defective (e.g. in longstanding RRDs of adults, particularly in myopia). In non-drainage surgery where break closure may take several days the surgeon should not be tempted to intervene if the buckle is seen to be appropriately positioned and of adequate dimensions. Closure of the break and subsequent absorption of the remaining SRF can be confidently expected to occur. Occasionally absorption of SRF may take an unexpectedly long time even when the break is apparently completely sealed. In these circumstances complete absorption of residual SRF may take several weeks and the temptation to inject gas into the vitreous cavity to hasten absorption should be resisted in most cases.

SRF absorption
<ul><li>SRF usually absorbs rapidly after break closure</li><li>SRF is sometimes delayed in spite of break closure – be patient</li><li>Failure to absorb or reaccumulation of SRF indicates failure</li></ul>

Proliferative Vitreo-retinopathy

Response of PVR to Conventional Surgery

- Regression. If PVR is not advanced and the membranes are still weak closure of retinal breaks and retinal reattachment will result in membrane regression. Post-operatively the membranes are scarcely detectable.
- Progression. When membranes are extensive and advanced simple closure of the retinal breaks, even if this can be achieved will not result in complete retinal reattachment. Tangential traction from membranes may prevent complete reattachment and the residual detachment (tractional) may become localised and non-progressive. More often the membrane formation continues and breaks are sequentially reopened and rhegmatogenous retinal detachment recurs.

PVR and Cryotherapy

Cryotherapy can cause the release of pigment epithelial cells into the vitreous cavity via the retinal break. These cells have the metaplastic potential to contribute to the formation of peri-retinal membranes. This should make the retinal surgeon wary of the injudicious use of cryotherapy. Usually however, the very cases which are more likely to lead to PVR (e.g. re-operations, blood in the vitreous and difficult retinal breaks) are precisely those in which there is a tendency to apply extensive cryotherapy. The potential contribution of cryotherapy to PVR has led to a more extensive use of laser retinopexy in vitreo-retinal surgery.

Early Anterior Segment Complications

- Sterile uveitis
- Infective endophthalmitis
- Ischaemia
- Closed angle glaucoma
- Open angle glaucoma.

Sterile Uveitis

Uveitis is found to a varying degree following most types of retinal detachment surgery, but least detectable after a non-drainage procedure. The degree of uveitis is increased with the complexity of the intraocular procedure or if complications (e.g. vitreous haemorrhage) have occurred.

Action

Anti-inflammatory therapy either as drops or systemic administration are effective in reducing post-operative pain and inflammation.

Infective Endophthalmitis

Intraocular infection is extremely rare, but is occasionally seen particularly following long and complicated intraocular procedures. It usually appears from a few days to 2 weeks after surgery. A previously quiet eye becomes red and painful and intraocular signs include an increase in flare and cells in the anterior chamber with hypopyon formation, and the vitreous becomes hazy.

Action

Prevention is important with concentration on aseptic theatre technique and the use of prophylactic antibiotics, given as a subconjunctival injection at the end of surgery. Treatment of endophthalmitis, if suspected, is the same as any other intraocular infection, i.e. a vitreous biopsy should be carried out and intravitreal antibiotics (eg, vancomycin 2 mg and ceftazidime 2 mg) injected (Chap. 20).

Ischaemia

Anterior segment ischaemia occurs as a result of reduced perfusion of the anterior segment and arises either from a reduction of arterial inflow from the anterior and long ciliary arteries or obstruction to the venous drainage by the vortex veins. Encircling procedures in compressing the whole globe are more likely to produce ischaemia than local buckles.

Mild anterior segment ischaemia is characterised by slight corneal oedema with inflammatory reaction in the anterior chamber and segmental atrophic iris changes many be seen. In severe cases there is thick flare and cells with marked iris atrophy, the iris assuming a somewhat greenish tinge with subsequent posterior synechiae, hypotony, and eventually cataract formation.

Action

Prevention is by far the best way of avoiding these problems. Appreciation of this problem has lead to a reduction in the use of encircling elements (particularly if high) and not detaching ocular muscles. Encirclement procedures should be avoided in any high-risk patient, e.g. in those with a general haematological problem such as HBSC disease.

Glaucoma

Closed Angle Glaucoma

This is rare and may occur as a result of:

- An anterior shift of the lens-iris diaphragm induced by buckling procedures (usually encircling). This type of glaucoma comes on within 24 hours of surgery and may be prevented by avoidance of high buckles in eyes that have predisposition to angle closure.
- Serous choroidal detachment. Associated detachment of the ciliary body may cause the latter to hinge forward on the scleral spur with shallowing of the anterior chamber and risk of angle closure.

Action

1. Pre-operative awareness of a shallow angle.
2. Medical treatment such as the systemic administration of Diamox and topical use of timolol 0.25% bd and Trusopt 2% bd will usually be all that is necessary to control the intraocular pressure until there is spontaneous resolution.

Open Angle Glaucoma

Open angle glaucoma is often seen following the more extensive types of vitreo-retinal procedures. It may be secondary to uveitis, and less commonly secondary to extensive vitreous haemorrhage (haemolytic glaucoma). Sometimes no obvious reason for a high pressure can be found but it is more likely to occur in eyes where there is underlying aqueous outflow obstruction, e.g. in patients with underlying chronic simple glaucoma.

Action

Usually systemic acetazolamide and local hypotensive agents (e.g. timolol 0.25% bd or Trusopt 2% bd) are all that are necessary to control the problem, which will resolve spontaneously in the weeks following surgery.

Early Posterior Segment Complications

- Choroidal detachment
- Vitreous haemorrhage
- Post-operative complications of intravitreal air.

Choroidal Detachment

Choroidal detachment may be serous or haemorrhagic.

Serous Choroidal Detachment

These occur in the first 48 hours following surgery, but their appearance may be delayed up to a week. They are smooth, dome-shaped elevations which may or may not be in direct relationship to the buckle (Fig. 11.1). They may be localised to one quadrant or involve the entire peripheral fundus. The elevations themselves have a brownish colour and although the fluid within them does not shift, the elevations have a wobbling movement. Posterior extension does not extend behind the equator and anterior spread tends to push the peripheral retina and ora serrata into view. There is almost invariably detachment of the ciliary body with hypotony. Choroidal detachments usually absorb spontaneously within a few weeks after surgery. Factors found to increase the likelihood of such detachments are vortex vein interference (due to cryotherapy or needle damage), myopia and drainage of SRF. Small choroidal detachments are insignificant and disappear spontaneously within a few weeks, with no tendency to jeopardise the outcome of the procedure. However, extensive choroidal detachments involving the greater part of the fundus can contribute to failure by increasing post-operative

If post-operative pain is severe consider:
- Infective endophthalmitis
- Glaucoma
- Severe anterior segment ischaemia

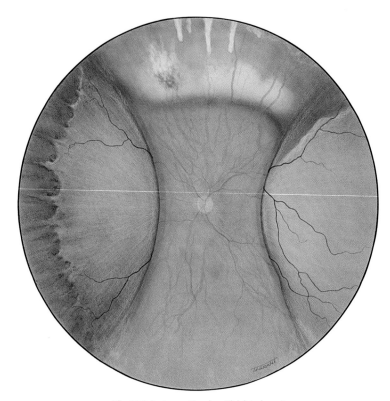

Fig. 11.1. Post-operative choroidal detachment.

inflammation and promoting PVR. If choroidal detachment is slight it leaves no evidence of its presence after absorption. If, however, it has been extensive there is often some degree of pigmentary disturbance taking the form of thin concentric lines conforming to the outline of the detachment.

Action

Usually none is required as the detachments will disappear spontaneously. Intraocular inflammation should be controlled.

Haemorrhagic Choroidal Detachment

This rare event arises almost invariably as a result of an operative choroidal haemorrhage and is often associated with some degree of overlying serous retinal detachment. Usually choroidal haemorrhage will spread into the subretinal space and into the vitreous cavity via retinal breaks and obscures the retinal view. The presence of blood within the eye greatly increases the chance of the eye progressing to PVR.

Action

An expectant policy should be pursued as in most of these cases choroidal haemorrhage will absorb spontaneously. However, if the haemorrhage is extensive then after 2 weeks further surgery should be considered, particularly if retinal detachment is present. This consists of external drainage of the choroidal haemorrhage (lysis of blood clot will have occurred), and PPV carried out. Silicone oil is usually injected. The prognosis is poor.

Vitreous Haemorrhage

This is a serious complication as blood in the eye obscures the retina and promotes PVR. Vitreous haemorrhage usually arises as a result of extension of a per-operative choroidal haemorrhage, although may be caused by rupture of a retinal vessel (e.g. caused by needle damage during SRF drainage).

Action

If the retina is obscured, B mode ultrasonography is necessary to establish that the retina is in place. If this is so, then an expectant policy can be pursued. However, if retinal detachment persists, then PPV should be carried out urgently to clear the vitreous haemorrhage and to secure the retina.

Post-Operative Complications of Intravitreal Air

Air is a soluble gas and is absorbed from the vitreous cavity within a few post-operative days. During this time observation of retinal details is more difficult.

Complications are rare:

1. Air may enter the subretinal space via large retinal breaks if injection technique has been poor and has resulted in multiple small bubbles.
2. Any intravitreal gas bubble tends to break down blood retinal barriers and induce some degree of post-operative inflammation, factors that may encourage the development of PVR. This is not noticeable in a short acting gas such as air, but it may be a contributory factor in the production of PVR if long acting gases (e.g. C3F8) are used in the non-vitrectomised eye.

Blood in the eye
Obscures retina and promotes PVR

Late Complications: Extraocular

Most extraocular complications following conventional retinal detachment surgery are related to the use of scleral buckles. These are:

- Cosmesis
- Explant extrusion and infection
- Pain and its causes
- Diplopia
- Refractive changes

Cosmesis

Low buckles cause almost no alteration in the appearance of the eye. Eyes that have had multiple procedures with loss of peri-ocular tissue (particularly those with high buckles) tend to be enophthalmic with consecutive ptosis.

Action

This condition is usually insufficient to require any corrective surgery, but if noticeable a lid elevating procedure may be necessary.

Explant Extrusion and Infection

Extrusion

Months or years after surgery there is a tendency for explants (particularly silastic sponges) to work loose and to assume a rather bulky swelling underneath the conjunctiva. Although not harmful, patients are often displeased by the appearance of such a lump. If the explant actually extrudes from the conjunctiva itself, it is likely that infection has played at least a part in this event.

Action

Explant extrusion is prevented by:

1. Meticulous suture technique using long intra-scleral sutures at the correct depth

2. Provision of a good covering of tenons and conjunctiva over the trimmed explant

3. Removal of explant may be necessary if the patient objects to its presence.

Infection

Silastic sponge is more likely to get infected than solid silicone, as are explants used at re-operations. (The incidence of infection is approximately 1%.) Although infection may manifest itself many months and sometimes years after surgery it probably arises as a result of low-grade infection introduced at the time of surgery. Infection takes the form of an extraocular syndrome – a mucopurulent discharge is produced from a dehiscence in the conjunctiva and this may be associated with granuloma formation (Fig. 11.2) and recurrent subconjunctival haemorrhage. The eye becomes red and irritable. On examination, care should be taken to elevate the lids and to move the eye into the extreme positions of gaze so that the infected areas may be brought into view.

Action

1. Prevention of infection is enhanced by the use of antibiotic-soaked sponges and subconjunctival injection of antibiotic at the end of surgery, and aseptic surgical technique.

2. An infected plant must be removed. Administration of antibiotics, either local or systemic, is ineffective. If a local explant is protruding through conjunctiva it may be gently grasped and pulled out after topical anaesthesia have been given. If the explant is buried or covered by granulomatous tissue removal is best performed under general anaesthesia. Provided the retina has been firmly attached and retinopexy around the breaks has been complete, the removal of explants will not result in retinal redetachment.

Pain

In the majority of cases pain encountered in the post-operative period is not severe and remits within a week or two of surgery. Sometimes, however, it may last for many weeks or even months, taking the form of a dull ache around the eye and referred to the side of the head in the distribution of the ophthalmic branch of the trigeminal nerve. Problems such as ischaemia, glaucoma, scleritis or uveitis may be the cause of such pain. However, on some occasions no intraocular problem can be demonstrated, the pain apparently caused by constriction from the scleral buckle. Such pain is much more likely to be encountered following the use of an encirclement procedure.

Action

Clinical examination will exclude ischaemia, glaucoma, scleritis or uveitis. If no positive cause can be found then simple analgesia (anti-inflammatory agents are helpful) will usually control the pain until it remits spontaneously. If this is not satisfactory removal of the buckle is necessary.

> Any patient with mucopurulent conjunctivitis following retinal detachment surgery should be suspected of harbouring an infected buckle. Infected explants must be removed.

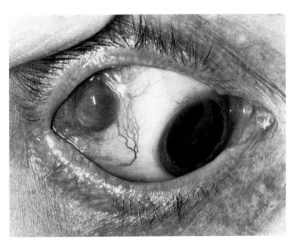

Fig. 11.2. Infection leading to a granuloma.

Diplopia

This has become uncommon as PPV is now preferred to deal with cases of difficult breaks (Chap. 15) which were previously treated by large and extensive buckles which tended to affect ocular motility. Transient diplopia occurs in about 5% of cases but the incidence of intractable diplopia considerably less. Muscle interference at surgery should be minimised and muscles should not be disinserted. The majority of cases particularly if image separation is not great settle spontaneously in a few weeks following surgery. Sometimes, however, diplopia may be intractable and this is particularly likely to occur if vertical diplopia is present.

Action

Prevention is achieved by:

● Avoiding muscle interference at the time of surgery
● Avoiding the use of unnecessarily large scleral buckles.

Treatment

Prismatic correction with spectacles may help, but if this is not satisfactory then squint surgery or botulinum toxin are advised. Simple removal of the explant will sometimes be helpful, particularly if this is not delayed for too long after retinal surgery has been performed.

Refractive Changes

Encircling Elements

When the buckle height is very low, refractive changes are minimal. If the buckle is somewhat higher, then there is a shift towards myopia due to elongation of the globe (up to 3 dioptres of myopia is common). With a deep encircling element the length of the globe is shortened with resulting hypermetropia.

Local Buckles

Minor degrees of change in refraction both of the astigmatic and spherical components are quite common following local buckling procedures. However, high deep local buckles, particularly if radial, may produce very substantial and lasting degrees of astigmatism (3 to 4 dioptres is not unusual).

Action

Most refractive errors following retinal surgery may be corrected by altering the spectacle correction (it is wise to wait for at least 2 months following surgery as there may be some alteration in the refractive status during this time). On occasions unacceptably high degrees of refractive error, particularly if astigmatic, may necessitate removal of the buckle some months after surgery.

Late Complications: Intraocular

● Macular changes
● Intraocular extrusion of explant
● Sympathetic ophthalmitis.

Macular changes

Macular Pucker

Macular pucker due to the presence of contracting pre-retinal membrane at the macula, is an unusual complication of all forms of retinal detachment surgery. (Incidence is approximately 5% of cases.) This incidence is higher in cases that already had established PVR (Fig. 11.3). The changes begin with disturbance of the normal macular reflex and wrinkling of the internal limiting membrane (cellophaning). The developing membrane is initially invisible but eventually thickens to form perceptible whitish tissue on the surface of the retina, neighbouring blood vessels become distorted and drawn into the centre of the membrane. The posterior hyaloid is usually detached. Intraretinal white dots, small haemorrhages, and later small exudates may be found together with serous fluid under the neuro-epithelium.

The clinical spectrum is variable. The condition usually commences about 6 weeks after surgery and

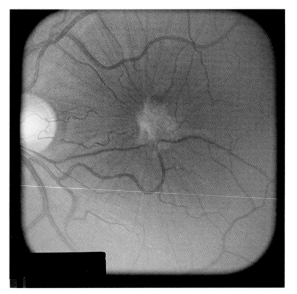

Fig. 11.3. Macular pucker following retinal detachment surgery.

Action

Mild cases with few symptoms and preservation of good central vision do not need treatment and are often non-progressive. Highly symptomatic patients need surgical treatment by PPV and peeling of membrane.

Other Macular Changes

Changes at the posterior pole following successful reattachment of the retina in cases in which the macula was detached occur occasionally. They may be non-specific pigment epithelial changes – with pigment epithelial proliferation and interspersed areas of atrophy, cystoid macular oedema (infrequent), or full-thickness macular hole formation (rare).

the reduction of central vision is accompanied by micropsia and metamorphopsia. In mild cases pucker is slight and reduction of central vision minimal. More usually reduction of central vision is substantial reducing the initial post-operative level of acuity by several lines. When occurring in an eye in which the macula was not detached prior to surgery the effects on vision are particularly devastating. Even in those cases where central vision is relatively good the patient may be considerably troubled by the incapacitating symptoms of metamorphopsia. Macular pucker of some degree occurs much more frequently in cases in which the retinal detachment had involved the macula in the pre-operative period, suggesting that the present of subretinal fluid under the macula tends to encourage the proliferative process.

Intraocular Erosion of Explants

This is now rare. Occasionally eroding materials (such as encircling elements or retaining scleral sutures) may result in recurrent vitreous haemorrhage which although disturbing usually clear spontaneously and require no active treatment; rarely retinal detachment occurs.

Sympathetic Ophthalmitis

This is rare complication of all forms of vitreoretinal surgery.

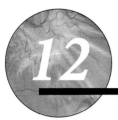

12 Rhegmatogenous Retinal Detachment: Failure of Conventional Surgery

Permanent retinal reattachment for cases of RRD uncomplicated by advanced PVR should be achieved with one operation in approximately 85%–95% of cases. If further surgery is necessary, this success rate should increase to over 95%. Failure of an operation is disappointing for both surgeon and patient and requires determination and understanding from both. It is particularly frustrating when initial visual improvement due to partial or complete absorption of SRF is followed by rapid worsening of vision due to redetachment. Careful explanation and prompt management will reduce the risk of a loss of confidence of the patient. Repeat surgery is not only more complex than primary surgery, but results from re-operation are worse both visually and anatomically. Failed surgery, particularly if complicated (e.g. by haemorrhage), tends to promote PVR making reattachment more difficult.

Behaviour of SRF

Non-absorption or progressive re-accumulation of SRF indicates failure of the operation. If SRF absorption is really complete it is unusual for the case to subsequently fail. The behaviour of SRF in the case of an inadequately sealed or missed break will depend on the type of operation performed.

- Failure after non-drainage surgery. In these cases SRF absorption will be incomplete, and its distribution will either remain unchanged if the original break is unsealed or will alter its distribution to conform to the position of an undetected break. Failure will usually be obvious 1–2 weeks from operation.
- Failure after surgery with drainage of SRF (e.g. D-ACE). In these cases the retina appear to have been almost completely reattached, only to be followed by progressive re-accumulation of SRF from an unsealed break.

The Reasons for Failure

The reasons for failure are:

1. Unsealed breaks (missed or inadequately treated) (Figs. 12.1, 12.2)
2. Proliferative vitreoretinopathy (PVR)
3. New breaks.

Unsealed breaks are the commonest reason for failed RRD surgery

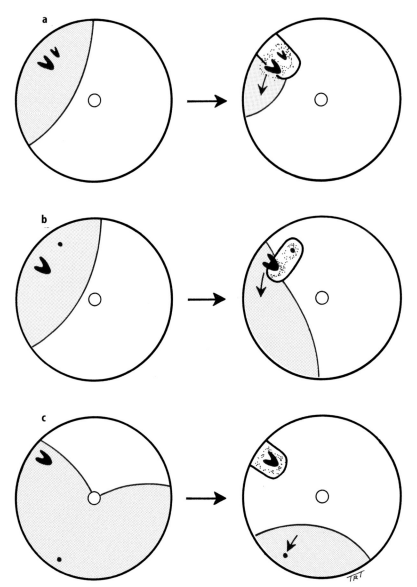

Fig. 12.1. Failed situations: **a,b** inadequate buckling; **c** a break in inferior retina has been missed. Note how the contour of the SRF changes to indicate the position of the missed break.

Unsealed Breaks

- Missed breaks. The failure to treat a break usually implies that the break has escaped detection
- Inadequately buckled breaks. A break may not be sealed because of:
    i.   Inadequate proportions of the buckle (insufficient height or width)

    ii. Poor selection of the direction of the buckle
    iii. Failure to close a break at surgery when there is local PVR even when a buckle of adequate proportions has been used.
- Inaccurate retinopexy. If retinopexy has been inadequate, but the break has been adequately buckled, redetachment of the retina may occur if the buckle height diminishes in the weeks or months following surgery.

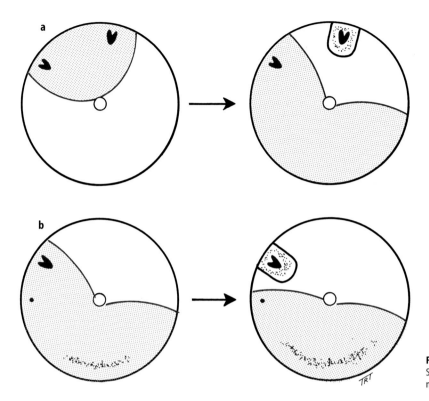

Fig. 12.2a,b. Breaks have been missed. The SRF distribution reflects the position of the missed break.

Proliferative Vitreo-Retinopathy (PVR)

PVR usually complicates rather than initiates failure and thus PVR will readily appear when retinal detachment surgery has failed to seal all retinal breaks. Apart from complicating failed cases in which there was no pre-operative PVR, PVR may be associated with failure in the following circumstances (Fig. 12.3).

1. When PVR is established prior to surgery (e.g. Grade C) it may progress after surgery in spite of apparent adequate break closure. This may even happen when PVR is less advanced (Grade B) but is much less likely (Fig. 12.4).

2. Rarely, PVR may suddenly develop several weeks after apparently successful surgery even when it had not been present at all in the pre-operative detachment state.

Action in Failed Cases

A full re-examination is carried out to establish the cause of failure and to enable a plan for further surgery to be made. Break detection is more difficult in the previously operated eye. Previous retinopexy reduces the contrast from the choroid in addition to which access to the break with scleral indentation is more difficult due to the presence of buckles, a difficulty that is compounded if the eye is sore and uncomfortable.

New Breaks

Rarely following complete reattachment of the retina a fresh break may occur months or even years after reattachment. These breaks are usually attended by fresh symptoms of vitreous detachment and such an event may be explained by extension

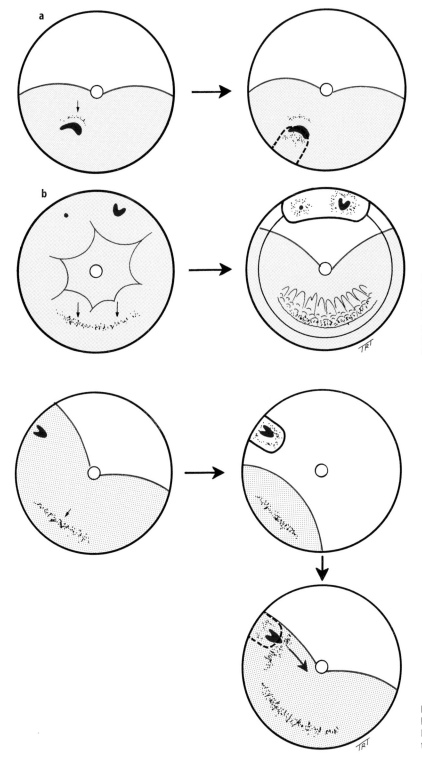

Fig. 12.3. PVR and failure. In **a** epiretinal membrane central to the break (*small arrow*) has prevented its closure. In **b** superior breaks have apparently been closed by surgery but inferior PVR has progressed to fixed fold formation. There is almost certainly an unseen and unsealed inferior break.

Fig. 12.4. An unusual cause of failure. The break has apparently been sealed but inferior PVR has progressed and eventually reopens the previously sealed break.

of what must have previously been an incomplete posterior vitreous detachment.

Choice of Surgery

Unsealed Breaks

Further Buckling

Re-operation will usually consist of a further buckling procedure, of either a previously unseen break or replacement of an inadequate buckle. Further retinopexy will be applied. The previous guidelines for non-drainage of SRF or SRF drainage and air injection or for PPV will be followed.

Gas Injection

In the unusual circumstance when failure has been caused by a break in superior retina which is slightly elevated from, but accurately sited over a buckle, it may be possible to achieve break closure with an intravitreal injection of an expanding gas (0.5 ml of 100% SF6) (Fig. 12.5). Post-operative posturing will allow tamponade of the break and additional retinopexy with laser photocoagulation is usually required after 24–48 hours. It is stressed that this is not often necessary as spontaneous closure of the break will usually occur without further surgical intervention.

Failure to Find Unsealed Breaks

In these cases management should be as described in Chap. 9 and surgery would thus consist of either presumptive buckling if the position of the unseen break is obvious or of PPV if more extensive detachment is present.

PPV

If failure has been accompanied by a rapid advance or appearance of advanced PVR (Grade C) then PPV and internal relief of traction will be necessary.

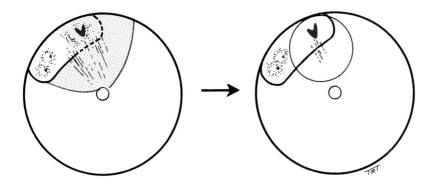

Fig. 12.5. The use of a post-operative gas bubble to seal a retinal break correctly sited over the buckle.

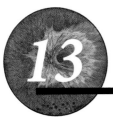

13 Rhegmatogenous Retinal Detachment: Prophylaxis

The object of prophylaxis is to prevent retinal detachment. Study of this subject has been neglected and as a result too many patients (approximately 50%) present with retinal detachment which has involved the macula. In many of these patients premonitory symptoms preceding the onset of the retinal detachment have been ignored either by the patients or unappreciated by those from whom the patient first seeks advice. In considering the need for prophylaxis, a balance has to be struck between the need to prevent detachment against the risk, necessity and economics of treatment. The consideration of an eye for treatment mainly concerns those conditions which are known precursors of retinal detachment, i.e. retinal breaks and those retinal degenerations which may lead to retinal breaks. Sometimes 'normal retina' is treated in high-risk eyes.

Retinal Breaks

The relative frequency of retinal breaks detected at post-mortem examination (about 5%) or noticed on routine examination (almost 6%) indicates, that as retinal detachment is a relatively infrequent occurrence (about 1 in 10 000 people each year) breaks only infrequently cause retinal detachment. It is necessary therefore to try to determine which breaks need treatment. Some types of breaks are more likely to cause detachment than others:

- Type. Retinal tears (with active vitreo-retinal traction upon their anterior aspect) are more likely to cause retinal detachment than round holes.
- Position. Breaks within the vitreous base do not to cause detachment (except retinal dialysis).
- Size. Big breaks are more likely to cause detachment than small ones.
- Myopia. Breaks are more likely to cause detachment in the myopic eye.

Symptomatic and Asymptomatic Breaks

If a break caused by a recent symptomatic PVD (floaters or flashes or both) is going to proceed to RRD then it will usually do so within a few weeks. After that time the risk declines (see Chap. 3 for presentation and symptomatology of PVD). Asymptomatic breaks, accidentally discovered, which may have been present for a long time, are less likely to cause detachment. However, patients are often relatively vague about symptoms so that the distinction between the symptomatic and asymptomatic eye, and therefore timing of the appearance of the

113

> Retinal breaks are the precursors of retinal detachment. It is better to err on the side of treatment rather than lose the opportunity of preventing retinal detachment.

retinal break may be difficult. Although some breaks carry a low risk of retinal detachment compared with others, it is still not possible to forecast with certainty which breaks will cause RRD and which will not. For example, on some occasions breaks of long standing may proceed to RRD. Urgent examination of patients with symptoms suggestive of posterior vitreous detachment should be carried out as soon as possible. Delay risks losing the opportunity of treating a retinal break prophylactically before it leads to retinal detachment.

Prophylactic Treatment

Prophylactic treatment of retinal breaks is advised in the following circumstances:

- Symptomatic breaks. Patients presenting with symptoms suggestive of posterior vitreous detachment and who are found to have a retinal break are at risk of developing retinal detachment, and all such breaks should be treated.
- Breaks in the high-risk eye. In these eyes the chances of a break proceeding to retinal detachment is greater than usual and breaks should be treated:
  i. Breaks in fellow eyes of patients with retinal detachments
  ii. Breaks in pseudophakic or aphakic eyes
  iii. High myopia.
- Breaks in asymptomatic eyes. All dialyses and retinal tears are treated, but small breaks within the vitreous base or if surrounded by retinal pigmentation indicating a longstanding nature do not require treatment.

Retinal Degenerations

It is important to establish which retinal degenerations risk break formation and which do not.

Benign Peripheral Lesions

All of these lesions are found in the equatorial and pre-equatorial regions of the retina. The absence of overlying vitreous abnormalities contributes to the benign way in which these lesions behave, i.e. full-thickness break formation does not occur. These lesions (Fig. 13.1) include:

- Choroido-retinal degeneration
- Choroido-retinal atrophy (paving-stone)
- Snowflake degeneration
- Cystic degeneration
- Pigment clumping
- White with or without pressure
- Retinal erosion.

Choroido-retinal Degeneration

The various types of choroido-retinal degeneration and the variations in their clinical appearance are harmless, widespread and non-progressive. Choroido-retinal degeneration is found in the retina immediately adjacent to the ora serrata, its appearance varying with its severity. When mild the only detectable change is a whitish-grey appearance on the surface of the retina with some degree of mottling and pigmentation. When more marked, the changes assume a more opalescent appearance with an increase of pigmentation and later peripheral arterioles are sometimes seen to be whitened and there is marked hyperpigmentation of peripheral retina. Choroido-retinal degeneration in the equatorial region takes the form of rounded elevated lesions with hyperpigmented borders or of a honeycombed area of pigmentation with the pigment tending to collect along the retinal blood vessels in a fine lace-like manner.

Choroido-retinal Atrophy (Paving-Stone Degeneration)

This degeneration is found in the equatorial and pre-equatorial regions and is characterised by the appearances of punched-out areas of retina with hyperpigmented borders. The lesions are usually linear in configuration, the centre of the affected

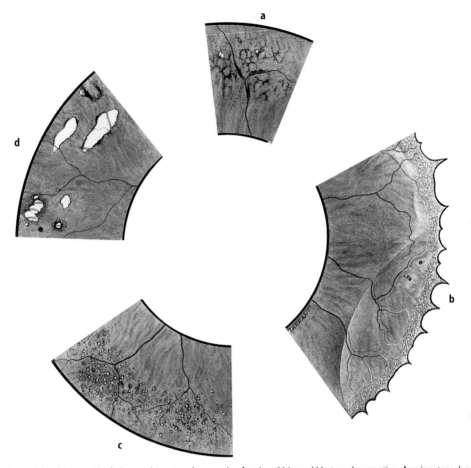

Fig. 13.1. Benign peripheral degenerative lesions: **a** pigmentary degeneration; **b** retinoschisis; **c** cobblestone degeneration; **d** paving stone degeneration.

areas varying according to the degree of atrophy present from either pink in mild cases to extreme whiteness when only bare sclera is apparently visible at the bottom of the lesion. However, in most cases larger choroidal vessels can be seen traversing the white areas. The overlying retina with the exception of the pigment epithelium which is absent, is found to be normal. It is not unusual to find extensive lesions which may, on occasion, extend through 360° of the peripheral retina. However, the lower half of the retina is usually favoured and the condition is bilateral. The lesions themselves although harmless and not leading to retinal break formation, may make detection of retinal breaks more difficult if retinal detachment is coincidentally present. Detached retina will always be adherent to the edge of the paving-stone areas.

Snowflake Degeneration

Snowflake degeneration consists of scattered yellowish dots, often multiple and close together in the postoral and equatorial region of the retina.

Cystic Degeneration

This degeneration begins in the outer molecular layer of the retina and results in the formation of cystic spaces in the neuro-epithelium. When these cavities coalesce and enlarge so that actual elevation of the retina can be observed the term retinoschisis is used. In its mildest form, cystoid degeneration is found immediately posterior to the ora serrata, the lower temporal quadrant being the most favoured. Pink-red vesicles on a whitish-grey background give an opalescent appearance, and on scleral depression the affected tissue assumes the appearance of fine frog-spawn. Occasionally the cystic cavities may rupture to produce small excavations mimicking retinal breaks. Cystoid degeneration is commonly found in eyes that show other forms of degenerative change. If extensive, this degeneration may extend towards but not posterior to the equator.

Pigment Clumping

A localised area of pigment clumping in the peripheral fundus is frequently seen; these areas are usually distributed between the ora serrata and the equator. The clumps are of no particular significance and are more often found in myopia.

White With and Without Pressure

These changes are seen in flat retina with or without scleral depression respectively. White without pressure is probably just a simple exaggeration of white with pressure. The condition is distinguished from the normal blanching of the choroid that comes about with scleral depression and which, accordingly, moves as the scleral depressor alters its position. In both conditions, geographical areas are found in the periphery of the fundus. The more linear edge of the area is on the ora serrata side of the lesion and the geographical shape on the more central side. Remarkably these areas extend posteriorly towards the equator and even beyond. The upper temporal quadrant is favoured and this appearance is often found in association with changes such as cystoid degeneration and lattice degeneration. These areas have not been shown to progress to any type of retinal degeneration of a more serious nature and may therefore be regarded as ophthalmic curiosities rather than areas of much significance.

Retinal Erosions

These are oval-shaped excavated areas within the vitreous base. The margins of such areas may appear to be slightly elevated and the base cratered in appearance. Small whitish tags of vitreous are seen in most cases. These areas are not associated with retinal break formation or retinal detachment, but are often seen in eyes that contain lattice degeneration.

Lesions That May Predispose to Retinal Detachment

These lesions may be associated with break formation, breaks that are either round holes due to retinal atrophy or retinal tears caused by vitreous traction.

- Lattice degeneration
- Snail track degeneration
- Cystic retinal tuffs.

Lattice Degeneration

In its typical form lattice degeneration consists of a sharply demarcated circumferentially orientated lesion located in the equatorial or pre-equatorial retina (Fig. 13.2). Typically the lesions may be seen in the second decade but are rarely progressive. The areas may be multiple and at different levels and the upper temporal quadrant is the most favoured. Bilateral lesions are found in about 50% of cases and even though present from an earlier age, the lesions are not often noticed until the fourth or fifth decade during an ophthalmic examination. The fine white lines pathognomonic of lattice degeneration are continuous with retinal blood vessels, which may be found emerging apparently quite normally on the

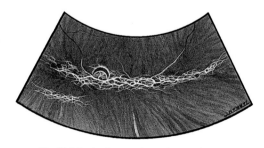

Fig. 13.2. Lattice degeneration with retinal breaks.

Lattice and snail track degeneration
• Often bilateral
• Equatorial
• Upper temporal quadrant is favoured
• Breaks may occur

anterior side of the lesion. The white lines, caused by hyalinisation of the retinal blood vessels, are associated with thinning of the neuro-epithelium although the choriocapillaris is itself relatively unaffected. Vitreous abnormalities overlying the lesions are frequent, with areas of adhesion interspersed with areas of liquefaction. The retina in the vicinity of lattice degeneration may have a somewhat thin and shaggy appearance, white dots are often found and there is a pigment epithelial reaction that varies in response from complete absence to extensive clumping. Retinal breaks are the most significant clinical features of lattice degeneration and they may be:

1. Round holes, in which case they tend to favour the ends of the lattice lesion.
2. Retinal tears, which are produced by posterior vitreous detachment and adhesion of gel to the posterior aspect to lattice. When a break is formed the lattice lesions are seen in the operculum.
3. Giant breaks occasionally but rarely arise from the posterior edge of a long section of lattice degenerative change.

As with retinal breaks the high incidence of lattice degeneration noted at autopsy (about 6%) in otherwise normal eyes renders it impractical and unnecessary to treat all patients with this condition. However, lattice degeneration, by leading to break formation, is a known precursor of retinal detachment. It occurs in approximately 30% of detachment cases, but not all of these cases are retinal breaks that cause the detachment associated with the lattice areas. The treatment of lattice degeneration is advised in the following high-risk situations:

- When breaks are found within it
- In the same or the other eye of patients with retinal detachment
- In aphakic or pseudophakic eyes.

Snail-Track Degeneration

Snail-track degeneration is so named because the lesions consist of sharply demarcated areas that have a glistening frost-like appearance and resemble the trail made by a snail (Fig. 13.3). The equatorial region of the retina is favoured, the changes are often bilateral and the temporal quadrant is affected most often. Although there are overlying vitreous abnormalities of liquefaction and adhesion, the breaks that are produced with this type of degeneration are round holes which may be quite large. Although tears do not occur there is a strong tendency to retinal detachment with this condition. Myopia is often present. Although this condition bears some similarity to lattice, and, indeed, it may just be a variation of it, hyalinisation of blood vessels is not seen and the two types of degenerations are not found together. Snail-track degeneration is less common than lattice.

Treatment

All round retinal breaks should be treated within the areas of snail-track degeneration. It is not necessary to treat the whole snail-track area.

Cystic Retinal Tufts

These are relatively insignificant small elevations in the post-oral region of the retina. If posterior vitreous detachment tractional breaks may arise at the posterior aspect of such tufts.

Treatment is not advised unless symptomatic retinal breaks occur.

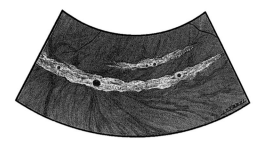

Fig. 13.3. Snail-track degeneration with round holes.

Retinoschisis

Retinoschisis may be classed as

1. Senile
2. Juvenile
3. Tractional.

Senile Retinoschisis

Senile retinoschisis originates from peripheral cystoid degeneration of the retina. These cystoid cavities become confluent in the outer plexiform layer. The retinoschisis thus formed progresses by extending in a posterior direction through the layers of the neuro-epithelium. The innermost layer of the schisis nearest the vitreous cavity is referred to as the inner leaf and the other leaf nearest the pigment epithelium as the outer leaf. Sometimes the cystic spaces enlarge to produce dome like elevations.

The main clinical features of this condition are:

- It is usually bilateral, occurring more in hypermetropic eyes, and the lower temporal quadrant is the most favoured.
- Yellow-white dots are scattered on the inner surface of the schisis cavity, apparently lying at the level of the internal limiting membrane. These dots are non-specific and may be found in other conditions, e.g. lattice degeneration.
- The inner leaf of the schisis has a beaten metal appearance seen on slit-lamp examination and retro-illumination.
- There may be sheathing or obliteration of overlying peripheral vessels.
- Retinal breaks are infrequent but may be found in the outer or inner leaf of the schisis and occasionally both. Breaks in the inner leaf are always round, whereas those in the outer leaf, which are difficult to detect, particularly at their posterior borders, can have a scalloped appearance, the edges of which are rolled. These breaks are usually irregular in shape.
- Demarcation lines are not seen and this helps distinguish retinoschisis from longstanding retinal detachment.
- Scleral depression over the outer leaf of the schisis makes the depressed area appear white. This is not seen in cases of retinal detachment.

- If retinoschisis extends posterior to the equator, an absolute field defect corresponding to the area effected is found.
- Vitreous haemorrhage is rare.

Clinical Course

Senile retinoschisis is either static or progresses slowly and cases in which the schisis extends towards the posterior pole are extremely rare. The great majority of patients with retinoschisis have no symptoms and suffer no visual loss and the condition requires no treatment. Occasionally retinoschisis cause RRD.

Management

The condition requires no treatment and patients do not need to be followed. Rarely retinoschisis may be complicated by RRD, which will need surgery.

Senile retinoschisis
- Usually bilateral
- Variable in extent and development
- No demarcation lines
- Rarely progressive
- Rarely causes RRD

Juvenile Retinoschisis

Juvenile retinoschisis is inherited as a sex-linked recessive disease affecting males or less commonly as an autosomal recessive disorder. The retina splits at the nerve fibre layer and the condition may be complicated by retinal detachment. The age of onset of this condition is usually less than 20 years. The affected retina has a thin cystic appearance and often multiple holes are present in the inner leaf. Early in the disease changes of retinoschisis are present in the macula as well, but they disappear in later life.

Management

No treatment is advisable. If retinal detachment occurs the prognosis for reattachment is poor.

Tractional Retinoschisis

Shearing forces on the retina caused by static vitreo-retinal traction (e.g contraction of vaso-proliferative tissue as in diabetes) can result in either tractional schisis if the layers of the retina are affected without separation from pigment epithelium or in tractional detachment if such a separation has occurred. Clinical distinction between these conditions does not appear to be important, but the features of tractional schisis are:

- Spread is slow
- Water marks do not occur (unlike tractional retinal detachment)
- Breaks may form in the inner leaf but do not result in rhegmatogenous detachment
- The edge of the schisis, where it meets normal retina, is convex towards the centre of the schisis, as in traction retinal detachment.

Management

No treatment is required for tractional schisis.

Methods of Prophylactic Treatment

- Treatment of second eye
- Technique
- Out-patient prophylaxis

> Do not miss the chance to detect asymptomatic disease – always examine the other eye

Treatment of Second Eye

As part of a retinal detachment procedure the opportunity to examine the second eye, particularly if general anaesthesia is to be used, should never be lost. Although, in the majority of cases the opportunity for prophylaxis will have been realised as a result of the pre-operative examination, occasionally undetected pre-operative pathology will become obvious on examination under anaesthesia. Transconjunctival cryotherapy or indirect laser photocoagulation is used. Serious complications are extremely rare with either method and there is little to choose between them. Conjunctival and lid swelling is avoided by using laser photocoagulation.

Technique (Fig. 13.4)

When small retinal breaks are treated the cryoprobe is placed directly underneath the break and usually only a single application of cryotherapy is necessary to freeze the retina around the break. With larger breaks, several applications will be needed. When linear areas are treated the cryo probe indents the centre of the lesion to freeze retina on either side. If it is necessary to treat extensive areas indirect laser photocoagulation is advised, not only to avoid lid swelling, but it is also easy to

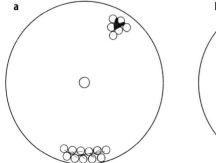
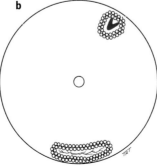

Fig. 13.4. a Cryotherapy surrounding a retinal tear and holes in lattice degeneration; **b** laser photocoagulation used for the same lesions.

see where the treatment is being applied so that areas to be treated are not missed. When laser photocoagulation is used two rows of treatment should be placed around the lesion to be treated. The actual laser spots should be close together, but not quite touching. The prophylactic treatment of the second eye of a patient with a giant break should consist of three rows of pre-equatorial indirect laser photocoagulation through 360° of retina.

Out-Patient Prophylaxis

Most lesions needing treatment may be treated with laser photocoagulation, and this can be done with the three-mirror contact lens with topical anaesthesia on a slit-lamp argon laser delivery system. This method will not always enable the most anterior aspect of a retinal break to be treated and this may be reached with either indirect laser ophthalmoscopy using scleral depression or by transconjuctival cryotherapy. If the latter is to be used a small subconjunctival injection of 2% lignocaine is required to achieve anaesthesia. On rare occasions some patients are quite unable to accept prophylaxis under local anaesthesia, and a general anaesthetic may have to be employed.

Serious Complications

Serious complications of prophylaxis are extremely rare. Macular pucker following the prophylaxis of retinal breaks occurs occasionally (there is no difference in the incidence of this complication between laser and cryotherapy) but it is difficult to know if the pucker had been produced as a result of treatment or consequent to the preceding posterior vitreous detachment.

Prophylaxis indicated
• All symptomatic breaks
• All breaks in fellow eyes of patients with RRD
• Other asymptomatic breaks (e.g. retinal dialysis and breaks and holes in lattice or snail-track degeneration, and most large breaks)
• Some lattice and snail-track degeneration even when breaks are not present
• 'Normal retina' in the fellow eye of an atraumatic giant break

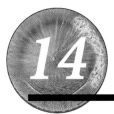

14 Pars Plana Vitrectomy (PPV): Basic Set-up

Good optics for visualisation of the posterior segment is an important part of the basic set-up of PPV. Systems for viewing through the operating microscope employ direct and indirect optics (Fig. 14.1).

Direct Viewing Using Contact Lenses and the Optics of the Operating Microscope

Traditionally, the posterior segment is viewed through the operating microscope using irrigating contact lenses during vitrectomy. A range of contact lenses is available with aspheric optics to give wide-angle or magnified central fundus views. These lenses are hand-held and require an attentive assistant with a steady hand to maintain a good view. The image produced is virtual and erect, the depth of focus is poor and the field of vision is small. The view of the peripheral retina is limited and prismatic lenses act as a mirror for visualisation of pre-equatorial retina. In gas-filled phakic eyes bi-concave lenses are needed to obtain a fundal view. These lenses can also be secured onto the surface of the cornea by retention rings that are held in place by sutures. Methylcellulose or visco-elastic agents are used as optical coupling agents. The retention rings hinder rotation of the globe and extreme movements often lead to displacement of the lenses by the lids. Bi-concave lenses have large prismatic effect and can produce displacement or distortion of the image if the alignment is not perfect.

Indirect Viewing Systems Using Image Inverters and Contact and Non-contact lenses

Many surgeons now favour indirect viewing systems using high-powered contact or non-contact lenses. A real and inverted image is produced which is then converted to an erect image by an image inverter incorporated into the microscope optics. The main advantage of an indirect viewing system is that it provides wide angle of viewing and a good depth of focus. There is no need for lens changes during gas/fluid exchange procedures. It is less dependent on pupil size and a good fundal view can be obtained even when the pupil is relatively small. Because the field of view is wide, there is less need to rotate the globe to see peripheral retina. When non-contact lenses are used, the cornea requires intermittent wetting and water splashing on the non-contact lens can spoil the view. Methylcellose

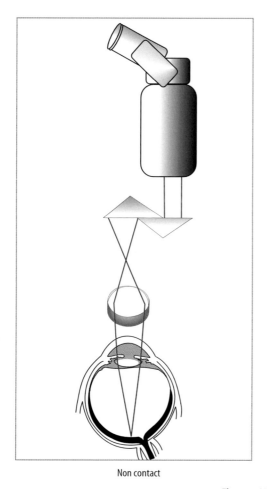

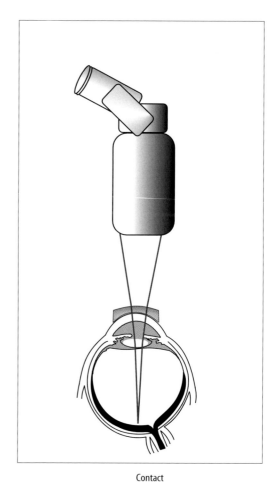

Non contact

Contact

Fig. 14.1. Viewing system optics.

or sodium hyaluronate can be used to wet the cornea and is particularly useful if the corneal epithelium has to be removed.

PPV

The operation of PPV has a number of features that are common to all operations involving this technique; these are:

- Anaesthesia
- Conjunctival dissection
- Muscle slings
- Sclerotomies
- Infusion fluid and pressure
- Optics for viewing the vitreous and retina
- Endo-illumination, vitreous cutter and other intraocular instruments
- Basic vitrectomy techniques including deep indentation and internal search
- Inspection of the retina for entry site tears
- Closure.

Direct viewing with contact lens and microscope optics	Indirect viewing with image inverter using contact lens or non-contact lenses
• Require an attentive assistant to maintain a good fundal view • Hands-free focusing is possible using the optics of the microscope and the foot control • Small field of view • Poor depth of focus • Need to swap lenses for the gas exchange procedure • Better for macular surgery?	• Wide field of view • Excellent depth of focus • Good view through small pupils • Requires an image inverter • Some systems require manual focusing • No need to change lenses for gas exchange • No damage to corneal epithelium

Anaesthesia

The choice of anaesthesia depends on:

• The anticipated duration of surgery
• The capacity and willingness of the patients to undergo local anaesthesia.

Local anaesthesia is becoming more popular and has, as a main advantage, a faster turnover of cases. Anaesthetists favour local anaesthetic because there is less risk of systemic morbidity in patients with medical history such as diabetes mellitus and cardio-pulmonary disease. Some surgeons prefer general anaesthesia as the duration of surgery is often unpredictable. This is particularly so in a teaching vitreo-retinal unit where training surgeons are usually slower than their more experienced tutor. General anaesthesia also allows a relaxed examination of the second eye with careful scleral indentation and examination that may not have been as satisfactorily performed in the pre-operative period. This examination will facilitate break detection and prophylaxis.

Most patients find the operations disconcerting and uncomfortable if the duration of surgery exceeds an hour and a half. Several of the surgical steps, such as cryotherapy and scleral indentation, can be painful if the local anaesthesia is inadequate or wearing off. Good akinesia is necessary for fine surgery close to the macula.

Whether general or local anaesthesia is used, the fitness of patients needs to be considered. Heart failure, uncontrolled diabetes mellitus or hypertension needs to be treated and such treatment should take precedence over elective surgery. Patients who have poor hearing, reduced intellectual power or who are highly anxious are best given general anaesthesia as a good degree of rapport between surgeon and patient to achieve co-operation and reassurance is essential when local anaesthesia is used.

For local anaesthesia, a 50%–50% mixture of 0.75% marcaine with 2% lignocaine with 1500 IU of hyalase is used. To achieve lasting akinesia and anaesthesia, our current practice preference is to use retro-bulbar anaesthesia in a single trans-conjunctivally injection in the lower temporal fornix using a 1-inch 25-gauge needle. The fornix is a useful landmark for the equator of the eye. A needle advanced antero-posteriorly at this site will have passed the greatest diameter of the globe and after about 1 cm the tip of the needle is directed superiorly, posteriorly and medially to ensure the injection is deposited inside the muscle cone. Balloting the globe with the shank of the needle as it changes direction gives a useful feel for the relationship between the globe and the tip of the needle. An injection of 6 ml of anaesthetic solution accurately placed in the retro-bulbar space provides up to $1^{1}/_{2}$ hours of good analgesia and akinesia. After 1 hour, it may be necessary to supplement the anaesthesia with repeated injections or topical anaesthesia as appropriate. For simple vitrectomies (i.e. those that will not involve scleral buckle or otherwise take more than 1 hour) retro-bulbar anaesthesia may be achieved by use of a curved cannula introduced into the sub-Tenon's space in the inferior nasal quadrant and slid round the contour of the globe. Approximately 3 ml of local anaesthetic may be injected in this way. Midazolam intravenously (1–2 mg followed by increments of 0.5–1 mg if not adequate, usual range 2–7.5 mg) can be helpful to anxious patients.

Conjunctival Dissection

A 360° conjunctival peritomy is necessary if scleral explants are planned or if deep scleral indentation is intended. Temporal and nasal relieving incisions aid exposure of the sclera overlying the pars plana. For a simple vitrectomy, it is sometimes only necessary to perform two fornix-based conjunctival flaps in the upper nasal quadrant and in temporal quadrant. Tenon's capsule should be reflected with the conjunctiva to reveal bare sclera around the sclerotomies.

Muscle Slings

Traction sutures around the rectus muscles facilitate scleral buckling procedures. They are unnecessary for simple vitrectomies.

Sclerotomies

For three-port vitrectomy, the infusion is sited over the pars plana in the temporal quadrant (Fig. 14.2). This is adjacent to the lateral canthus to give maximum room to rotate the eye during surgery. The sclerotomies are placed 4 mm behind the

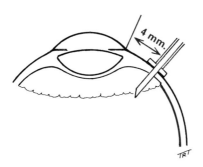

Fig. 14.2. The infusion cannula.

limbus in the fully grown phakic eye to ensure the eye is entered anterior to the vitreous base (to avoid making a dialysis) but this is sufficiently posterior to avoid damage to the crystalline lens. The sclerotomies are sited more anteriorly (3.5 mm from the limbus) in microphthalmic, aphakic and pseudophakic eyes. In the neonate, lens-sparing vitrectomies are possible with sclerotomies placed 1.5 mm behind the limbus. Diathermy over the sclera ensures haemostasis and the sclerotomies are usually made with micro-vitreo-retinal (MVR) blades. The blade is directed towards the disc to avoid damage to the lens. Following preparation of the sclerotomy, the infusion cannula (usually 4 mm in length) is inserted into the eye. After the cannula is inserted careful inspection will confirm that it has penetrated into the vitreous cavity. This can be done through the operating microscope by indenting the cannula deeply or with the indirect ophthalmoscope. The tip of the cannula needs to be visualised clearly before the infusion is turned on. Pre-placed sutures are used to secure the infusion cannula and may be tied as a bow.

Suture

This suture can be used to close the sclerotomy at the end of the operation when the infusion cannula is removed; 9/0 nylon or 8/0 Vicryl are generally used for the sclerotomies.

Special Note on Technique

Extra care needs to be exercised when operating upon eyes with suspected choroidal detachment. In presence of choroidal detachment, it is not sufficient to see the tip of the cannula on indentation, one has to ensure a large part of the shaft is inside the vitreous cavity. In these cases, the non-pigmented epithelium of the pars plana can hood over the cannula. Infusing under the detached non-pigmented epithelium will detach the choroid and sometimes the retina as the vitrectomy proceeds. If

> The infusion cannula must be fully within the vitreous cavity

there is hooding, a cut-down of the non-pigment epithelium from an adjacent port using an MVR blade should be made. It may also be appropriate to use a longer cannula (6 mm).

Where to Place the Upper Sclerotomies

The upper sclerotomies are made as horizontal as possible. This position allows easy access to pre-equatorial retina and pars plana without reaching across the posterior pole of the lens and risking lens touch. The sclerotomy is thus placed to give equal access to the upper and lower halves of the retina and is helpful when extensive anterior dissection is planned in cases of anterior PVR. Anterior/inferior foreign bodies may also be removed from horizontal ports. If the nose hinders the movement of the instruments when the nasal port is in the horizontal meridian the sclerotomy has to be slightly higher in this quadrant.

The MVR blade produces a 20-gauge slit. It is often difficult to introduce square-ended instruments through a linear opening. The slit can be rounded up by a Nettleship punctum dilator or a 20-gauge needle, thus facilitating the introduction of awkwardly shaped instruments.

Extra steps which are helpful in deep set eye include:

- An anterior chamber infusion cannula can be used in aphakic eyes instead of a standard pars plana infusion
- Retro-bulbar anaesthesia to displace the globe forward
- Gentle traction on rectus sling muscles has the same effect
- A simple wick to prevent welling up of irrigation fluid in the fornix.

Complications of Sclerotomies

1. Haemorrhage. Slight intraocular haemorrhage may occur. If so, this is usually insignificant.
2. Too large. If the sclerotomies are inadvertently made too large, then leakage of intraocular contents, either infusion fluids, gas or liquid silicone can be a nuisance making it difficult to maintain the intraocular pressure. This is more likely to occur at re-operations when previous sclero-

tomy sites may be accidentally reopened. If this problem becomes anything more than a slight nuisance, the sclerotomy site may have to be completely resutured and a fresh site selected.
3. Breaks. Manipulation of the vitreous base may result in retinal dialysis. Traction on the posterior hyaloid at the time of instrument entry and exit into the eye may produce small retinal tears.
4. Extrusion of vitreous (and retina) may occur if sclerotomy sites are left open and intraocular pressure is high.

These complications are usually only encountered when there has been excessive manipulation of the sclerotomy sites from awkwardly shaped instruments (such as scissors) and will not occur during simple vitrectomy instrumentation (such as use of cutter, light pipe and flute needle). When there is a risk of breaks, careful inspection of the sclerotomy sites at the end of surgery is essential to recognise and treat any offending breaks.

Infusion System

The object of such a system is to retain a steady intraocular pressure during surgery preventing hypotony and collapse of the eye. Hypotony risks choroidal haemorrhage, which is one of the worst complications of vitreo-retinal surgery. It may also result in bleeding into the anterior chamber and also induce folding of the cornea both of which can obscure the fundal view.

Infusion Fluid

Hartmann's (Lactated Ringer's) solution is usually used for infusion. Special Balanced Salt Solutions may have advantages in maintaining corneal and lens clarity for protracted vitrectomies. Adrenaline (1 ml of 1:1000 into a litre bottle of Hartmann's solution) may be added and this will help to maintain pupil dilatation.

Avoid per-operative hypotony

Bottle Height

The height of the infusion bottle should be adjusted to suit the conditions of surgery. Usually it is placed at about 30 cm above the eye to maintain intraocular pressure. If there is systemic hypotension, the arteries at the optic nerve head can be seen to be pulsating and the infusion should be lowered. Sometimes the disc is obscured as in cases of proliferative diabetic retinopathy. If poor perfusion is suspected, the bottle height should be lowered. Conversely, the height may be raised to achieve haemostasis briefly by raising the intraocular pressure during dissection of vascular membranes. If the bottle height is raised, care must be taken to keep sclerotomies closed for fear of extrusion of intraocular contents. The intraocular pressure is also determined by suction applied via the cutter and to the rate of leakage of fluid through sclerotomies.

Vitreous Cutters and Endo-Illumination

Most modern vitreous cutters are driven by pressurised air. The cutting rate can be 800 or higher per minute. The instrument is designed to excise vitreous gel piecemeal thereby exerting minimal traction on the body of the gel. Traction on the gel can give rise to retinal tears especially when the cutter is at the vitreous base. Usually, the maximum cut rate with a suction of between 150 and 300 mmHg is used for vitrectomy. When working close to the retina, the suction needs to be reduced. The cutter should not be moved around within the gel without cutting otherwise traction generated by the suction may cause retinal tears. Modern cutters all have a guillotine action with an inner shaft moving under an outer sleeve. The closure is achieved by air pressure and the opening by a spring. The whole instrument is light and the inertia is small. This means the rapid action of the cutter does not produce juddering movements of the whole probe inside the eye. Cutters with smaller ports close to the tip facilitate the cutting of tissues close to the retina.

Mode of Action

Virtually all vitreous cutters for posterior segment work are driven by the Venturi principle. Suction is generated by forcing air through a narrowing aperture. The increased velocity of the air produces negative pressure or suction. The suction is then applied via a chamber through a length of tubing and the cutter and into the eye. The chamber acts a reservoir for collecting vitreous fluid. The presence of this chamber means that negative pressure can be built up in the system, a fact that must be constantly be borne in mind when working close to the retina. Suction can continue even when the foot is off the pedal until the Venturi is vented. For this reason, most vitrectomy machines are designed with relatively small chambers and narrow-bore tubing to reduce the volume of the reservoir. Some machines have more than one chamber so that when the small reservoir is filled it is decanted to a larger reservoir for storage.

Priming of Cutter

It is generally unnecessary to prime the tubing as its volume is relatively small. This allows undiluted specimens of vitreous fluid to be collected for biopsies and microbiology. When the cutter is used for delicate dissection or closely applied to the mobile retina, the foot needs to be taken off the pedal frequently to vent the system of negative pressure.

Endo-Illumination

A halogen light source provides good illumination. Blunt-ended light pipes give a divergent cone of light and moving the endo-illumination probe further away from the object gives a wider field of illumination. The divergence is a result of refraction as the light passes from the higher refractive index of the fibre-optic into the vitreous fluid. The cone of illumination is therefore wider in air-filled eyes. The vitreous gel is best observed with the light directed perpendicular to the direction of viewing. The retina on the other hand is best seen by direct illumination. As a compromise, and in order to see both the vitreous and its relationship to the retina, the light pipe is held obliquely. In the course of a vitrectomy, the direction of the endo-illumination probe is constantly adjusted to give best visualisation of the structure of interest.

Tapered light pipes give an enhanced field of illumination and complement the wide-field optics of the indirect view system. The shape of the tip makes it easy to introduce the light pipe through sclerotomies.

Intraocular Instruments

A wide variety of instruments is available for each specific task. Many instruments are available for once-only use. The use of each instruments has to balance need against cost and most vitrectomies can be performed with a few basic instruments (e.g. a 23-gauge needle or an MVR blade can be bent at the tip to make a useful pick).

Of the many instruments available, the simple flute needle is indispensable. The simplicity of design relies on passive aspiration of fluid with the suction pressure governed by the height of the infusion pressure. Passive aspiration as opposed to active aspiration means that hypotony can be avoided. A bulb attached to the flute opening allows reflux of fluid. A jet of fluid can be used to agitate settled red blood cells and facilitate their removal. The flute needle enables the exchange of fluid for air, drainage of diffuse blood and occasionally allow direct manipulation of retina under silicone oil or heavy liquids. It helps de-laminate epiretinal membranes in cases of macular pucker. Some cannulas have a Portex tubing at the tip and thus are useful for identifying the posterior vitreous lamina in macular hole surgery.

There are many intraocular forceps and scissors available for intraocular surgery. Most are hand-held but some have a mechanised action. The blades of the scissors are available with different degrees of angulation allowing horizontal and vertical cutting actions, the most popular of which is 70°, which are often used for de-lamination of pre-retinal membranes in cases of proliferative diabetic retinopathy. These awkwardly shaped instruments can engage basal gel on entry and cause entry site tears. At the end of the operation, close inspection of the pre-equatorial retina adjacent to sclerotomies using deep indentation is mandatory to detect and treat breaks.

There are now many instruments that have more than one function built into 19- or 20-gauge systems. For example, a multi-function probe is available with endo-illumination, aspiration and diathermy facility. These instruments allow more complicated manoeuvres to be carried out without repeatedly changing instruments.

Complications

- Infusion: choroidal or retinal detachment from infusion fluid
- Sclerotomy site: breaks, haemorrhage, extrusion of vitreous or gel
- Instruments: lens touch, retinal breaks
- Anterior segment: corneal oedema, hyphaema, intraocular lens difficulties.

Air Infusion

A continuous air infusion pump is used for exchanging intraocular fluids with air. It may be a separate piece of equipment or be incorporated as part of modern vitrectomy machines. The preset pump pressure is not equal to intraocular pressure and hypotony is possible. The intraocular pressure depends on achieving a steady state, when the rate of infusion of air keeps up with the rate of leakage of contents from the eye. During air infusion the flute needle is maintained in fluid behind the enlarging air bubble. If fluid exchange is done using active or passive aspiration, the rate of evacuation of fluid may exceed the air infusion and hypotony ensues. Similarly, when an eye is air-filled it may leak rapidly through an open sclerotomy venting the system to the atmosphere. Fluctuations in intra-ocular pressure occur when instruments are removed from the eye but should be kept to a minimum by keeping sclerotomies closed as much as possible.

Basic Vitrectomy Techniques (including deep indentation and internal search)

Routine Checks

A routine of checks should be made before the commencement of the vitrectomy; ensure that:

- The infusion cannula is in the vitreous cavity
- The correct infusion fluid is being used
- The infusion bottle height is not too high
- The cut-rate and suction pressure are correct
- The microscope is set up to allow a comfortable operating position.

Vitrectomy can involve lengthy and complex manoeuvres. Both surgeon and the scrub nurse should be aware of the intended surgical moves so as to avoid unnecessary delay during the procedure.

The basic vitrectomy uses endo-illumination and a vitreous cutter (Fig. 14.3). The angle and the penetration of the light probe is varied to give optimum illumination. At all times there must be awareness of the spatial relation between the vitreous cutter and the back surface of the crystalline lens. Tilting and rotating the eye excessively will alter the relative position of the cutter and may cause lens touch. In

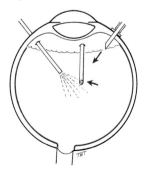

Fig. 14.3. The standard three-port vitrectomy set up with infusion cannula, fibre-optic illumination and vitreous cutter.

phakic eyes, all intraocular instruments should be directed at post-equatorial retina.

The opening of the cutter, which must be visible to the surgeon at all times, should be rotated to face the vitreous gel it is cutting. Ideally, vitrectomy should start at the posterior vitreous face (provided this can be identified) and continue anteriorly leaving a small residual frill at the retina. Repeated insertion of the instruments should be minimised to avoid risk of entry site breaks.

Deep Indentation

This technique is of basic importance to the performance of vitreo-retinal surgery and its importance cannot be over-emphasised.

Indications

- Clearing of anterior vitreous opacity
- Identifying retinal breaks
- Assisting the dissection of anterior pre-retinal membranes

Deep indentation is useful for clearing peripheral opacities (e.g. blood), identifying retinal breaks and enhancing removal of peripheral gel and sometimes anterior pre-retinal membranes. It should be used to complete an anterior vitrectomy.

Clearing Vitreous Opacity

Technique

This procedure should be done with the bottle height reduced to render the eye compressible. Indentation may be performed as a bi-manual technique and for this a shortened squint hook hook serves as a convenient scleral depressor. This instrument is used to indent the globe bringing peripheral retina into view and allows access of the vitreous cutter to the gel frill. This move can be carried out by the surgeon using the coaxial illumination of the microscope, the indentor in one hand and the vitreous cutter in the other. This technique is useful for removing vitreous opacity such as blood in anterior inferior gel. However, better illumination may be achieved by indentation from an assistant leaving the surgeon free to use endo-illumination and vitreous cutting. To avoid lens touch in the phakic eye, the nasal port should be used for anterior vitrectomy of the nasal half of the eye and the temporal port for the temporal half. Lens touch is also minimised by avoiding excessive tilting of the eye. Indentation is facilitated by suction from the vitreous cutter, otherwise firm pressure on the globe will raise intraocular pressure and risk incarceration of vitreous or retina into either an open sclerotomy or the infusion cannula. When the latter happens, the infusion stops flowing and hypotony ensues often for a period before the surgeon becomes aware of the situation. Similarly, care should be taken when using the technique of deep indentation in the presence of a highly elevated retina which may incarcerate into any of the ports.

Break Detection

Deep indentation allows inspection of the vitreous base to search for vitreous breaks (see Chap. 15, Fig. 15.1). The light pipe is inserted through one port to illuminate anterior retina and a plug is inserted in the other unused port. Using endo-illumination, an excellent view is achieved which is free from the specular reflection of the cornea and lens. The mobility of the depressor backwards and forwards across the vitreous base brings into view retinal breaks undetected before surgery.

Drainage of SRF

Deep indentation can assist the drainage of SRF. A scleral depressor indents under the break and the vitreous cutter trims the gel around the base of the break. With linear aspiration, a large proportion of the SRF can be evacuated, especially if the fluid is viscous, as when the retinal detachment has been present for a few weeks. (The drainage of SRF in this way is less successful for fresh detachment as the retina surrounding the retinal break tends to become quickly apposed to the pigment epithelium loculating the bulk of SRF posteriorly.) As soon as SRF is drained, air exchange needs to be carried out promptly otherwise infusion fluid rapidly recruits through the break. This is facilitated by maintaining scleral indentation and when air is introduced into the eye, the cutter continues to aspirate close to the break. As soon as the air fills the anterior part of the vitreous cavity the break is effectively sealed, the indentation can be released and both light pipe and a draining flute needle inserted to complete the pre-retinal fluid/air exchange. Evacuation of SRF using deep indentation cannot be expected to achieve a complete drainage. Slight residual SRF will be displaced posteriorly and there is a danger of driving SRF underneath the macula, which may not have been detached prior to surgery. To avoid this complication complete air fill should be avoided (see Chap. 15).

Deep indentation: the dos and don'ts
• Indentation can be performed by the surgeon (as a bi-manual technique) or by an assistant
• Reduce bottle height and infusion pressure
• Deep indentation is enabled more by aspiration than by pressure
• Prevent lens touch by avoiding tilting the eye or reaching across the posterior pole of the lens in phakic eyes

Retinopexy

Retinopexy following vitrectomy is carried out with laser photocoagulation or with cryotherapy. For small areas to be treated there is probably little to choose between the two methods. Laser photocoagulation has some advantages, but is not without technical difficulty.

The advantages are:

• It is less likely to promote PVR
• It causes less discomfort and swelling postoperatively
• It probably causes chorio-retinal adhesion earlier than cryotherapy.

Viewing Difficulties

Laser photocoagulation is usually delivered via an endo-probe and occasionally via an indirect ophthalmoscope. Laser retinopexy is only possible when the retina is apposed to the underlying pigment epithelium and although retinal apposition can sometimes be achieved with indentation alone, this is usually only possible for anything but small breaks after fluid/air exchange. However, small breaks may then be difficult to visualise through the air bubble. The treatment of posterior retinal breaks (including retinotomy sites for SRF drainage) usually presents no difficulty. If a retinal break is situated in pre-equatorial retina, deep indentation using a bi-manual technique is needed to get access. The view through an air bubble using the coaxial illumination of the operating microscope is less satisfactory.

This viewing problem is overcome by the multi-function light probe that incorporates two fibre-optic fibres, one carrying endo-illumination and the other carrying the laser. It offers the surgeon the freedom to carry out deep indentation with one hand, whilst illuminating the break and treating at the same time using this probe in the other hand. An alternative method to overcome the viewing difficulty is to carry out laser retinopexy by first re-apposing the retina with heavy liquids. Using the wide-view optics afforded by an indirect viewing system it is possible to gain access to the equatorial retina without the need for deep indentation. The uptake can be variable when the laser encounters multiple reflective and refractive interfaces between air and cornea, cornea and lens, lens and air and air and retina. Laser can be delivered via an indirect ophthalmoscope combined with scleral indentation.

> Treat small breaks before fluid/air exchange

Cryotherapy

If a limited amount of retinopexy is required, cryotherapy may be used and this can achieve retinopexy even if a shallow film of SRF is present and can therefore be applied before fluid/air exchange. Cryotherapy is performed either in the conventional manner using an indirect ophthalmoscope (with plugs in the sclerotomy port) or using the indirect viewing systems of the operating microscope. The latter is performed with the endo-illumination light probe inserted through one of the two sclerotomies, a plug in the other and using the cryotherapy probe as a scleral indentor. This provides good viewing of the retinal breaks before or after fluid/air exchange.

Inspection of Entry Site

At the end of a vitrectomy, the retina should be inspected for entry site breaks by indirect ophthalmoscopy or by deep indentation. This is best carried out before air exchange as break detection can be difficult in the air-filled eye.

Closure

The sclerotomies should be closed using 8/0 Vicryl or 9/0 nylon after any prolapsed gel has been carefully removed from the wound using the vitreous cutter. The wound should be sewn tight to prevent leakage of internal tamponade agent post-operatively. A drop of atropine 1% will maintain dilation of the pupil facilitating fundoscopy at the first dressing.

Long-term Complications

The most important long-term complication is the development of nuclear sclerotic cataract. In patients over the age of 50 this is an almost invariable complication about which the patient must be warned. In younger patients, the risk of cataract formation is greatly reduced. Cataract surgeons should be warned that absence of the vitreous from an eye gives it a rather 'soft' feel. Phacoemulsification and intraocular lens implantation may be used as usual.

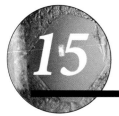

15 Pars Plana Vitrectomy: RRD without PVR

PPV proved to be an important addition to the choice of procedures available to the vitreo-retinal surgeon in the management of RRD. PPV should not just be regarded as a procedure to follow failed conventional surgery, but may well be the operation of first choice. Case mixes will be dissimilar between various centres but in our two units vitrectomy is performed as a first operation for RRD in 30%–40% of cases. The indications for PPV for RRD are separated into two groups:

1. RRD uncomplicated by significant PVR.
2. RRD complicated by PVR where the main reason for PPV is to solve the problems caused by the peri-retinal membranes.

PPV for RRD without Extensive PVR

In these cases vitrectomy is not being performed because of PVR and it is useful if the RRD is associated with any of the following features:

- Difficult breaks
- Macular pucker
- Choroidal detachment
- Foreign body.

Difficult Breaks

Breaks are classed as difficult because of:

- Uncertainty of position
- Size
- Position
- Arrangement

Detection Uncertain

If the view of the retina due to opacities in the media is completely or partially obscured, detection of retinal breaks may be either impossible or unreliable. The commonest causes of opacities are at the lens iris diaphragm (e.g. poor pupillary dilatation, cataract, opacification of the anterior and posterior capsules with or without residual lens remnants following cataract extraction or other forms of trauma) or because of vitreous opacity (e.g. vitreous haemorrhage). In the pseudophakic eye these difficulties are further compounded by awkward light reflection from the surfaces of the intraocular lens. The following characteristics of breaks make them difficult and potentially risky to buckle conventionally.

The Size of Break

Breaks greater than one clock hour in size (huge buckles would otherwise be required to seal these breaks).

Consider PPV as the operation of first choice

Position

Breaks at the posterior pole are inaccessible to easy buckling.

Arrangement

Multiple breaks widely scattered and of varying size and distance from the ora serrata that would otherwise demand a very complex arrangement of buckles. Multiple breaks of this sort may be found in 'ordinary' RRD or may be part of an exceptional picture such as retinal detachment complicating CMV retinitis.

In all of the above examples of 'difficult breaks' PPV allows safe internal drainage of SRF, controlled retinopexy and easy closure of breaks by internal tamponade. When breaks are situated above the midline use of buckles will be completely avoided (see later).

Macular Pucker

If macular pucker accompanies RRD then the visual result, which may be achieved following reattachment of the retina with conventional methods, will be disappointing due to the presence of the pucker. In these cases PPV combines peeling of the pre-retinal membrane with closure of peripheral breaks.

Choroidal Detachment

If choroidal detachment is extensive particularly if in close proximity to retinal breaks then PPV is advised. At least partial drainage of the supra-choroidal fluid will occur from the sclerotomy sites at the time of operation allowing for break closure and retinopexy.

Foreign Bodies

The presence of an intraocular foreign body which is judged to need removal.

Rationale for PPV

The rationale for PPV when PVR is not present in any significant degree is as follows:

1. Allows clearing of opacities in the media
2. Enables break identification
3. Removes dynamic vitreo-retinal traction upon breaks which can then be closed and sealed with internal SRF drainage, gas tamponade and retinopexy. This also reduces the need for scleral buckling.

Surgical Technique

- Removal of Anterior Segment Opacities
- PPV
- Break detection
- Internal drainage of subretinal fluid
- Retinopexy
- Fluid/air exchange
- Buckles
- Air/gas mixture

Removal of Anterior Segment Opacities

Significant cataract will be removed either by phacoemulsification (this is particularly useful if marked nuclear sclerosis is present) or via pars plana lensectomy. It may be possible to retain either anterior or posterior capsule to allow insertion of an intraocular lens at a subsequent operation. Opacities anterior to an intraocular lens (e.g. anterior capsule) will have to be removed with scissor dissection via a corneal incision. Cataractous remnants from previous congenital cataract surgery may be very difficult to manage. Tough doughnuts of almost calcified material may be present which will be difficult to remove with the vitreous cutter through the pars plana. These remnants may have to be removed with scissors dissection via a corneal incision. Visco-elastic material is extremely helpful when injected into the anterior chamber to clear blood or white cells which may obscure the view of the posterior segment. Intraocular lenses are retained whenever possible, removal only being necessary if they are judged to severely impair the view of the retina. Posterior capsular opacities are removed with a vitreous cutter via the pars plana sometimes after an initial incision into the capsule with the MVR blade has been made. If a plate haptic lens is present capsulotomy (if necessary) should be small.

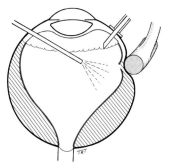

Fig. 15.1. Indentation is used to find peripheral retinal breaks.

PPV

In the presence of mobile retinal detachment the infusion bottle is kept low and high cutting rates are used to minimise the risk of the retina being sucked into the cutter and producing iatrogenic breaks and haemorrhage. Central vitreous is removed first until the posterior hyaloid is identified and this is then removed in a central to a peripheral direction until the point to which the vitreous is attached to the retina (usually but not invariably the vitreous base) is reached. A short frill is left at the point of retinal attachment. If the posterior vitreous detachment is very incomplete then this can usually be encouraged, if not always completely achieved, by gentle traction on the posterior hyaloid. This manoeuvre is more difficult to achieve in the young eye. The trimming of peripheral vitreous is facilitated by external indentation.

> Search detached and flat retina for breaks

Break Detection

Although large breaks become obvious as the vitrectomy proceeds, particularly if they are equatorial or post-equatorial in position a careful internal search is made to detect breaks in both detached and flat retina. The mixing of SRF emerging through a retinal break with infusion fluid (Schlieren) is of little localising value. During PPV retina that was previously flat will not usually detach and the distribution of SRF from retinal breaks is therefore still predictable. A careful internal search should now be made to now detect breaks in both detached and flat

retina. Internal searching with indentation and light pipe illumination allows a magnified binocular view of retina, a technique that is particularly helpful for the detection of small peripheral breaks (Fig. 15.1). Just as with scleral depression in the pre-operative examination the use of per-operative indentation affords an important dimension to the examination. Occasionally indirect ophthalmoscopy and external indentation may be useful, particularly if there is still some residual problem in peripheral visualisation while viewing with the microscope.

Internal Drainage of SRF

Internal drainage of SRF is achieved via the retinal break either with a flute needle tapered to 27 gauge for small breaks or using the vitreous cutter and low suction. In spite of this it may be difficult to evacuate SRF through small peripheral breaks.

Retinopexy

Cryotherapy applied through full thickness sclera or endolaser photocoagulation is used. If breaks are large and difficult to close with indentation then retinopexy can be delayed until after fluid/air exchange. All breaks both in detached and flat retina are treated. Laser photocoagulation is particularly simple and suitable for breaks which may be readily closed with indentation. If retinal breaks are small and easily closed it is wise to apply retinopexy before the fluid air exchange as the breaks may be very difficult to detect through the minified image afforded by the gas bubble. If breaks are large and if they are difficult to close at this stage then retinopexy can be delayed until after fluid air exchange. All breaks both in detached and flat retina are treated.

Fluid/Air Exchange

Air is introduced to the eye via the three-way tap on the infusion system. The indirect viewing system facilitates fluid air exchange as it requires little if any alteration in the focusing of the optical system. Fluid is removed with a flute needle from behind the enlarging intravitreal bubble (Fig. 15.2). SRF should be evacuated via a retinal break early in the exchange, otherwise the enlarging intravitreal bubble will close a peripheral break making the evacuation of subretinal space more difficult. After SRF has been exchanged and the break closed the tip of the needle is advanced into the eye until all fluid is removed from the pre-retinal space.

When gas is used as an internal tamponade, it is not necessary to chase the last residual drop of SRF. The success of surgery depends on the identification and closure of retinal breaks and any residual SRF will absorb as usual in the post-operative period.

Buckles

Post-operative gas tamponade will be perfectly adequate to achieve break closure for superior breaks until they are sealed by the retinopexy reaction (approximately one week). Tamponade however, of breaks below the mid-line is much less certain and buckling for equatorial and pre-equatorial breaks in

the inferior retina is recommended. These buckles (of silicone rubber) need only to cover the break and do not have to be high. The 287 tyre is satisfactory for most purposes. Encirclement is not necessary.

Air/Gas Mixture

Prior to closure of the sclerotomies, the eye is filled with the gas mixture to be chosen. Sulphahexafluoride (SF6) is particularly suitable for cases of RRD without PVR. A 20% air/SF6 mixture is suitable as it will not expand when introduced into the eye and will provide satisfactory tamponade of superior breaks for at least 10 days while it is gradually absorbed. This mixture is flushed through the eye via the infusion cannula and is performed manually using a 50 ml plastic syringe. If general anaesthesia is employed at which nitrous oxide is being used then the latter should be discontinued 10 minutes before the exchange. This is to ensure that nitrous oxide which is freely soluble is not part of the air bubble in the eye prior to the air/SF6 exchange. If this is not done there may be a rapid reduction in the size of the gas bubble after the nitrous oxide has been discontinued at the end of surgery.

Per-operative Difficulties and Complications

Complications which may be encountered at any PPV have been described in Chapter 14. Specific

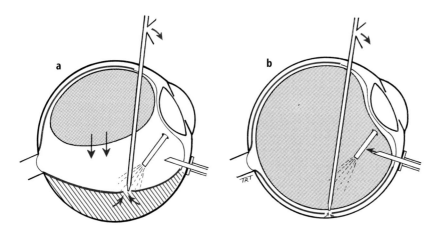

Fig. 15.2. Internal drainage of SRF via the retinal break as part of fluid/gas exchange.

difficulties and complications of PPV for RRD without PVR include:

- Retinal breaks
- Difficulty with break detection
- Difficulty with fluid/air exchange
- Choroidal haemorrhage

Retinal Breaks

Iatrogenic retinal breaks may be caused by the cutter and these have to be closed and sealed.

Difficulties with Break Detection

On some occasions in spite of assiduous per-operative searching, particularly in cases which have had previous operations the view of the extreme periphery may still be difficult. Absolute certainty about break detection may be impossible. Failure to find a retinal break is always very uncomfortable and leads to a series of presumptive moves based on the likely site of the unseen break.

Action

Retinopexy should be applied to all suspicious areas particularly concentrating on the suspected site of the retinal break. If retinopexy itself also fails to show up the site of a break then a small posterior retinotomy should be made using a 20 gauge endo-diathermy tip (approximately 2 disc diameters above the disc provided there is reasonably deep SRF) to allow internal drainage. A further search of peripheral retina should be made both before and after gas exchange to see if the alteration in the retinal configuration has revealed a break. If a superior break is likely then buckling is not required. If the retinal detachment is confined to the inferior half of the retina, the retinotomy should be equatorial in position, so that subsequent to drainage and gas exchange an inferior buckle can be used to seal both the retinotomy and also the presumptive retinal break. If the detachment is more complete and an inferior break can be excluded, then after drainage and gas injection buckling is unnecessary.

Difficulties with Fluid/Air Exchange

This may be caused by

- Pseudophakia
- Aphakia
- Small breaks

View lost?	
	Action
● Corneal oedema	Remove epithelium
● Folds in Descemet's	Restore IOP
● Ant. Chamber cells	Healon to AC
● Condensation on IOL	Flute wipe
● Specular Reflection from Bubble	Keep exchanging
● Vitreous haemorrhage	Raise bottle before aspiration

Pseudophakia

A variety of difficulties may arise in the pseudophakic eye. These include condensation on the back of the intraocular lens (the droplets usually quite easily removed by the flute needle) anterior displacement of the lens-iris diaphragm , shallowing of the anterior chamber causing displacement of haptics, or actual entry of air into the anterior chamber itself (which can severely obscure the view of the posterior segment). The latter problems may be dealt with by injecting visco-elastic material into the anterior chamber displacing air from it and pushing the lens-iris diaphragm backwards.

Aphakia

Miosis may be profound in spite of infusion of adrenaline or subconjunctival Mydricaine. Small sphincterotomies will have to be performed to enlarge the pupillary aperture, although iris hooks may be used.

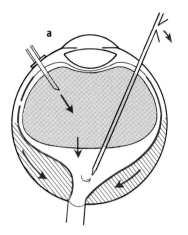 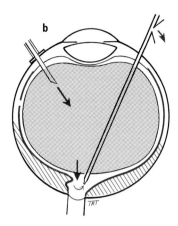

Fig. 15.3. Failure to evacuate SRF anteriorly may result in posterior movement of SRF as the gas bubble enlarges. Pleats may form in posterior retina.

Small breaks

If the retinal break is small it may be difficult to completely evacuate the SRF. If this is not possible enlargement of the air bubble in the pre-retinal compartment will tend push fluid in the subretinal space backwards towards the disc (Fig. 15.3). This steam rolling action not only risks detaching what may have been a previously un-detached macula, but may also result in retinal pleats. This problem may be avoided by;

1. Instead of attempting a complete air fill of the eye a bubble of 100% SF6 (1.5 mls) which will not caused posterior displacement of SRF may be injected into the vitreous cavity. This bubble will double its volume within 48 hours of surgery and can be relied upon to provide adequate tamponade for most superior breaks. Residual SRF will absorb spontaneously in the postoperative period.

2. A posterior retinotomy to evacuate SRF may be used. The retinotomy will be sealed with endolaser retinopexy after fluid/air exchange.

3. Heavy liquids when introduced into the eye will sink to the posterior pole and progressive filling of the eye will push SRF forward and out through peripheral retinal breaks. A heavy liquid/air exchange will then be performed.

Choroidal Haemorrhage

Severe per-operative haemorrhage is a rare but dreaded complication of PPV. It is more likely to occur if there have been periods of hypotony, or extensive retinopexy and buckling. The myopic eye is much more vulnerable to this complication. If choroidal haemorrhage occurs and is extensive, per-operative evacuation of the haemorrhage will rarely be successful and the eye will have to be closed. Although the prognosis for restoration of good vision is poor, after two or three weeks there may be an opportunity to re-operate, drain choroidal haemorrhage externally, and remove internally the almost inevitable accumulation of subretinal and vitreous blood. Silicone oil tamponade will usually be necessary.

Failed Surgery

Failure to completely achieve reattachment or re-detachment of the retina is due to failure to seal breaks at the time of surgery. In some cases appearance or advancement of PVR may contribute to the process of failure.

Failure to Seal Breaks

This failure may be because of:

- Missed breaks
- Unsealed breaks

An assiduous per-operative search for breaks both in detached and flat retina must be carried out. In clear media this is a simple task, but it is still difficult if there are residual opacities (e.g. IOL's and capsular opacities). The vitrectomised eye is unforgiving and missed breaks even in flat retina will cause redetachment much more readily than those in the unvitrectomised eye. Iatrogenic breaks made by the cutter during PPV will usually be obvious at the time of surgery, but breaks made at sclerotomy sites by the introduction of instruments are much less so.

Unsealed Breaks (Fig. 15.4)

Breaks may be unsealed due to:

1. Failure to surround breaks with retinopexy at the time of surgery (breaks that are small may be difficult to find after fluid/air exchange)
2. Retina may redetach from breaks deliberately not treated with retinopexy (e.g. macular holes)
3. If buckles have been used for inferior breaks then they must be placed accurately and of adequate dimensions to achieve break closure

4. If buckles are not used then correct posturing of the patient is as necessary to seal superior breaks. Occasional failures occur if patients are unable to co-operate with posturing requirements.

PVR

The incidence of PVR with redetachment in the vitrectomised eye is not obviously higher than that after conventional retinal detachment surgery. PVR complicates rather than initiates failure. On rare occasions apparently complete flattening of the retina with sealing of breaks may be followed by the rapid onset of PVR which may then reopen previously sealed breaks.

Clinical Presentation in Failed Cases

All patients having PPV for RRD without PVR are treated with gas tamponade as part of their opera-

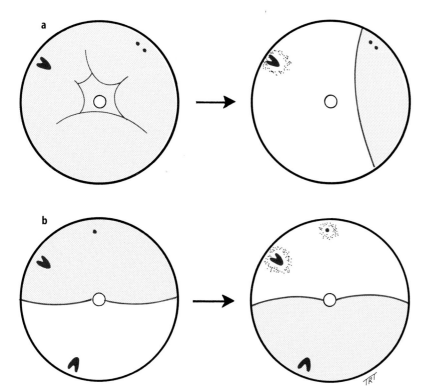

Fig. 15.4. Failed situations after PPV: **a** missed breaks in superior and previously detached retina; **b** break has been missed in inferior and previously flat retina.

tion. If breaks had been missed then retinal detachment will usually appear a short time after the absorption of the gas bubble (i.e., present within a few weeks of surgery). Sometimes redetachment is delayed for a surprisingly long time (months). If redetachment does occur SRF accumulation is usually rapid, and the site of the missed break will conform to the usual rules of SRF spread as in the non-vitrectomised eye.

The main symptom of retinal detachment in the vitrectomised eye is that of a rapidly spreading field defect and depression of vision if the macula becomes involved.

Management

A complete re-examination should be made to try to identify the unsealed break.

Choice of Surgery

1. Repeat PPV and gas tamponade. Pre-operatively it is often not possible to identify with certainty the site of the unsealed break (s) and therefore in most cases re-operation will consist of a further three port PPV approach with careful further internal searching for the offending break. When found internal drainage of SRF with gas tamponade and retinopexy is carried out. If PVR has appeared near the break or if the break is in inferior retina then scleral buckling of the break should be performed.

2. Pneumo-retinopexy. If it can be seen that failure has been caused by an unsealed break in superior retina, then this can be treated with a simple fluid/gas exchange under local anaesthetic. 1 ml of fluid is removed from the vitreous compartment and replaced with 1 ml of 100% SF6. This gas bubble will double in volume within 48 hours and retinopexy may be applied either in the form of cryotherapy at the time of surgery if the break can easily be reached or, laser or cryo retinopexy applied a few days later after break closure has been achieved.

3. Repeat PPV plus silicone oil. If extensive PVR has appeared then silicone oil will be necessary at re-operation (see Chapter 16).

Results

Anatomical success with one operation for RRD without PVR treated by PPV should be seen in about 85% of cases.

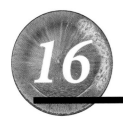

16 Pars Plana Vitrectomy: RRD with PVR

The surgery of RRD complicated by PVR presents some of the most demanding challenges in ophthalmic surgery, not only in the complexity of the surgical moves, but also in the art of weighing the visual and anatomical expectations of surgery against the likely benefit to the individual patient. Successful surgery may restore useful field of vision but in advanced cases detailed central vision is rarely achieved. The indication for the use of conventional scleral buckling to treat mild cases of PVR has been covered in Chap. 9.

Rationale of PPV

In addition to the advantages of vitrectomy discussed in Chap. 15 for cases of RRD without PVR, when PVR is present vitrectomy has some added advantages:

- It provides access to the retinal surface to remove epiretinal membranes and thus aid break detection, break closure and enable relief of traction.
- It removes cells and inflammatory material from the vitreous cavity
- It provides space for long-acting tamponade agents.

Vitrectomy is used when it is necessary:

1. To remove epiretinal membrane in order to reveal and achieve closure of retinal breaks
2. To remove epiretinal membrane in order to achieve retinal reattachment
3. To treat RRD complicated by macular pucker.

Surgery for PVR Cases: Initial Set-up

The basic set up for PPV has already been described (Chap. 14), but there are additional features to be considered in these highly technical and demanding cases:

- The use of binocular indirect viewing system
- Pupil dilatation
- Treatment of the lens.

The Use of Binocular Indirect Operating Microscope Viewing Systems

The availability of binocular indirect operating microscope systems has greatly enhanced vitrectomy for PVR. Such systems provide a panoramic fundal view and facilitate the dissection of anterior traction systems. This is particularly helpful for epiretinal membrane dissection when membranes are pulled away from the retina. It is essential to see the effect of such traction not only in the vicinity of the instrument but also to observe the pull on the retina remote from the site of surgery. Using deep indentation and a light pipe, it is possible to perform an internal search for retinal breaks in the pre-equatorial retina. The lack of specular reflection from the microscope light, the great depth of focus and the wide-angle viewing all enhances the chance of break detection.

Pupil Dilatation

The pupil may be miosed pre-operatively. This is usually either from previous surgery of the lens-iris diaphragm or from inflammation leading to posterior synechiae. Miosis may also occur per-operatively because of hypotony or manipulation of the iris. In these instances, restoring intraocular pressure and the addition of adrenaline one part per million (1 ml of 1:1000 adrenaline into a litre of Lactated Ringer's) in the infusion fluid will result in pupil dilatation in about 10–15 minutes. In spite of these simple moves the pupil may remain profoundly miotic.

Action:

1. Flexible nylon sutures
2. Sphincterotomies

Where the iris is atonic or fibrotic and the freed pupil is still small then pupil-dilating sutures can provide an excellent view. Flexible nylon single-use sutures are easy to use. Normally, four sutures provide excellent visualisation. Alternatively, it is possible to take small nibbles of the iris sphincter with the vitreous cutter to assist pupil dilation but broad iridectomy or complete extirpation of the

sphincter should be avoided. A permanent dilated pupil would allow silicone oil into the anterior chamber and result in oil keratopathy. Manipulation of the iris usually results in marked flare and proteinaceous exudation in the anterior chamber postoperatively. Pupillary membranes, posterior and anterior synechiae or pupil capture can form.

The Lens

It may be difficult to decide whether or not to remove the crystalline lens.
Advantages of removal:

- Facilitates vitreous base dissection
- Enhances the view in cases where there are lens opacities.
- Most lenses eventually become cataractous whether silicone or gas is used. Primary cataract removal obviates the need for subsequent cataract surgery.

Disadvantages:

- Pupil block when silicone is used (and oil keratopathy)
- Reduces the effectiveness of silicone oil as an internal tamponade
- The chance is missed for performing more controlled lens extraction at a later date, after the posterior segment has been stabilised.

An important aspect of PVR surgery is the dissection of the vitreous base. This can be accomplished with deep indentation in phakic eyes. With experience, it is possible to use instruments up to the ora without lens touch. However, the dissection is made easier when the eye is aphakic or pseudophakic. If the lens is clear and PVR is not so advanced that extensive anterior dissection is going to be necessary, the lens is left. However, if the case is more advanced, the lens is already cataractous and if it is anticipated that extensive anterior dissection is going to be necessary then lens extraction is advised.

Methods of Lens Removal

For removal of clear lenses, pars plana lensectomy via one of the sclerotomies is convenient. If a lens is sclerotic or frankly cataractous then phacoemulsification via a separate scleral tunnel is the method of choice. With both methods of lens removal, it is probably necessary to remove all the capsule if silicone oil is to be used to enhance the chance of patency of the inferior iridectomy that will be made.

In the pseudophakic eye, the posterior lens capsule in contact with silicone oil will become opaque. A wide capsulotomy should be performed.

Removal of Epiretinal and Subretinal Membranes

The management of the posterior segment is initially that of a routine vitrectomy, removing all the gel as far anteriorly as possible, i.e. up to the vitreous base. This is followed by the removal of epiretinal membrane and involves:

- Choice of using forceps and picks
- Obtain a starting edge
- Start beside larger blood vessels
- Work along valleys of fixed retinal folds
- Peeling: how deep to dissect and how hard to pull?
- The use of heavy liquid

Forceps and picks. Epiretinal membranes are engaged by forceps and gently pulled off the surface of the retina. This is particularly appropriate for starfolds as the membrane is thickest and easiest to purchase with forceps at its centre (Fig. 16.1). Picks are used if the dissection is unusually difficult. Picks are sharpened spatulas (sometimes incorporating endo-illumination) designed for lifting epiretinal membranes. A simple bent 23-gauge or MVR needle often serves the purpose equally well. Needles and picks are used to define a plane of separation between the epiretinal membrane and the retina.

Sometimes when the membrane formation is less obvious a plane of cleavage has to be established. This plane is often not apparent as the retina is translucent and it is difficult to judge the thickness of membranes. A good place to start the dissection is over blood vessels or within the valley of retinal folds.

Only experience teaches how hard to pull membrane without producing retinal breaks. The direction of the peel should be away from the surface of the retina. Older membranes are less cellular, more fibrotic, and less adherent to the underlying retina and are much more readily removed than younger membranes which are more diaphanous, difficult to engage and more adherent. Attempting to remove recently formed membranes is more likely to produce retinal breaks.

Dissection of anterior epiretinal membranes is difficult because of poor visualisation and access. The membranes are often an integral part of the vitreous base, which in normal circumstances cannot be detached from the retina. Working in a radial direction, it is possible to relieve the pursestring effect of membrane contracture at the vitreous base. Again, the bi-manual technique of deep indentation will enhance access.

Subretinal strands and membranes are elastic and seldom cause sufficient traction on the retina to require removal. Rarely, subretinal membranes are judged to produce irreducible fixation of the retina and if so then a retinotomy is made in the vicinity of one of the membranes which can then be gently grasped and pulled out.

The Use of Heavy Liquid for Peeling Epiretinal Membranes (ERM)

The per-operative use of perfluorocarbon liquids has been found to be of great value in assisting the surgery of PVR. It is useful:

- To open a tight funnel of detached retina
- To stabilise the retina for epiretinal membrane peeling
- To assess the relief of traction.

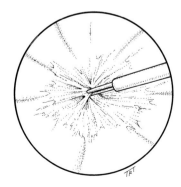

Fig. 16.1. A starfold is removed by grasping its centre.

In the case of the closed funnel, it is difficult to get access to the depth of the funnel to peel ERM. By introducing a small bubble of heavy liquid, the surface energy of the perfluorocarbon will open the cone and reveal circumferential edges to be purchased by a needle tip or a pair of forceps (Fig. 16.2). The dissection should be meticulous, working postero- anteriorly introducing incremental amounts of the heavy liquid. As the bubble of heavy liquid gets larger however, this surface energy decreases and its role in dissection of ERM is limited once the bubble exceeds about 1.5 ml (Fig. 16.3).

Heavy liquid also stabilises mobile retina for ERM peel. The retina is 'flattened' such that it is easier to apply a perpendicular pull upon the ERM without the fear of digging into the retina. The dissection of anterior ERM is greatly facilitated by rendering the posterior retina immobile with heavy liquid. This allows traction to be placed upon the retina to enable the anterior membranes to be dissected (Fig. 16.3).

The use of heavy liquid can also provide useful information on the extent of relief of anterior traction If the ERM removal has been effective, the retina will be re-apposed by the heavy liquid. If the retina remains elevated then there must still

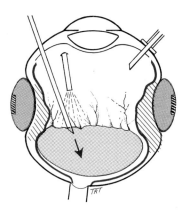

Fig. 16.3. Heavy liquid aids the dissection of epiretinal membranes.

be residual traction. Further dissection will be needed and possibly relieving retinotomy peformed.

Per-operative Complications of Heavy Liquids

Heavy liquid should be injected using a coaxial double cannula designed for the purpose. The heavy liquid passes into the eye through the central lumen and pre-retinal fluid escapes through the outer lumen, which has an opening near the tip of the cannula. Injection of heavy liquid using a single 20-gauge cannula raises the intraocular pressure and risks causing vitreous incarceration into a sclerotomy or the infusion cannula.

Heavy liquid in PVR
● Stabilises retina
● Improves access
● Relief of traction

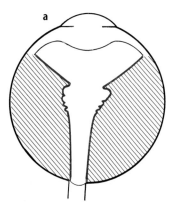
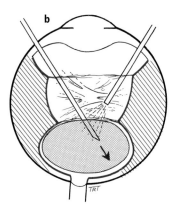

Fig. 16.2a,b. The use of heavy liquid to open a tight funnel of detached retina to reveal ERM.

The fill of heavy liquid should not extend beyond the most posterior retinal breaks when there is still unrelieved traction. If so, the surface tension of the heavy liquids may be overcome by the rigidity of the retina and further filling can cause the heavy liquids to overflow into the subretinal space. Attempts should be made to avoid rigorous intraocular currents caused by the infusion as they will break up the heavy liquid to form small bubbles which may find their way into the subretinal space via the breaks. The infusion bottle should be low. The tip of the injection cannula should be inside the enlarging bubble of heavy liquid at all times otherwise small bubbles will form.

Perfluorocarbon liquids should be removed completely at the end of operation with the flute needle to avoid potential retinal toxic effects. This is performed as part of a fluid/air or fluid/oil exchange.

Subretinal Heavy Liquid

When heavy liquid is used in cases of giant retinal tears or relieving retinotomies, small bubbles can be washed into the subretinal space by intraocular currents. These bubbles either singly or as a collection of several small droplets can cause shallow elevation of the retina. The appearance resembles frogspawn under the retina. They tend to gravitate to the posterior pole around the optic disc but can also be trapped at the edge of the retinal tear or retinectomy by an incoming silicone oil bubble. If left, a droplet of subretinal heavy liquid can settle under the macula post-operatively and give rise to a cystic appearance with damaging consequences to the recovery of central visual acuity.

Action

This is a complication best prevented by avoiding overfilling. Subretinal heavy liquid has to be removed either via a posterior retinotomy or it can be reached if a large peripheral retinotomy has been made.

Surgery for Giant Retinal Tear

It is appropriate to consider the surgery for giant retinal tears at this point as although PVR may not necessarily be present the surgery for these cases often involves techniques that are used in PVR surgery. All cases should be treated urgently due to the rapid onset of PVR that, in addition to the usual changes of PVR, result in scrolling and fixing of the posterior flap of the giant break.

The surgical sequence is:

- Removal of the vitreous gel especially anterior to the retina tear
- Unfold and stabilise the giant break which may require removal of any ERM to do so
- Retinopexy
- Injection of silicone oil

Vitrectomy

Most phakic giant retinal tears should be managed with a lens-sparing vitrectomy. After completing a posterior vitrectomy, deep indentation is used to trim the gel base. If a large amount of gel frill is left behind, it may prevent re-apposition of the retina to the underlying pigment epithelium. If the break is uncomplicated by PVR, then proceed to the injection of heavy liquid. The injection should start slowly at the posterior pole and the surface tension of the heavy liquid gradually unfolds and re-apposes the retina (Fig. 16.4). Even utilising the surface tension of the heavy liquid, it is not always possible to unfold a tightly scrolled large retinal tear and sometimes, it is necessary to gently stroke the retina to help it unfold. This can be done with the tip of the endo-illumination light probe although specially designed retinal 'brushes' or cannulae protected with portex tubing are available for this manipulation.

Removal of Epiretinal Membranes

If ERM are encountered these should be removed with forceps or picks. The direction of peel should be tangential to the retinal surface rather than perpendicular because pulling indirectly on the retina towards the centre of the vitreous cavity can result in the heavy liquid going into the subretinal space. The retinal tear is unfolded as far as possible. In advanced PVR, rigid pleats cannot be unfolded easily even after assiduous removal of epiretinal membranes. In this situation, retinectomy should be

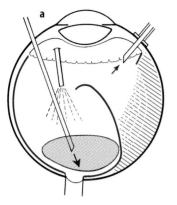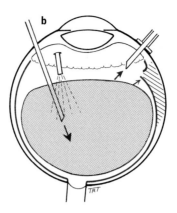

Fig. 16.4a,b. Heavy liquid is useful to unroll the posterior edge of a mobile giant break.

carried out sacrificing all rigid retina in order to get complete apposition of the posterior retina. A circumferential incision parallel to the ora made over the extent of the retinal tear is sufficient in some cases although more commonly there is also anterior PVR involving the other clock hours and a 360° retinotomy is needed. In exceptionally severe cases small radial relieving retinotomies may be needed to achieve retinal re-apposition.

Retinopexy

Once the giant tear is totally re-apposed, further injection of heavy liquid can safely be made as there is now no risk of the liquid entering the subretinal space. This will stabilise the whole retina in preparation for silicone oil exchange. Prior to exchange it is necessary to apply endo-laser to achieve retinopexy. Photocoagulation is carried out along the posterior edge of the giant retinal tear. It is not necessary to treat the anterior frill of isolated retina. Special attention needs to be paid to the two ends of the tear by ensuring the laser photocoagulation is extended anteriorly to the ora serrata. This can usually only be achieved with deep indentation and in a phakic eye access may be difficult. It is acceptable and expedient to use cryotherapy to ensure that the two 'horns' of the giant tear are properly treated. Although satellite breaks must be treated, it is uncertain whether or not the part of the retina uninvolved with the giant tear needs to be treated as there is apparently very little risk of subsequent break formation occurring in the vitrectomised eye particularly when silicone oil is used. If it is to be

done it is preferable to use laser retinopexy rather than cryotherapy.

Silicone Oil Exchange

Silicone oil is rarely used for RRD without a significant degree of PVR. Exceptions to this are cases which have a strong tendency to PVR formation (e.g. the giant break) or those in which the arrangements of the retinal breaks suggest that if gas tamponade was used there might be a risk of re-detachment in patients who are seriously ill (e.g. the retinal detachments associated with CMV retinitis where breaks are multiple, difficult to find and widely scattered). Long-acting tamponade agent is needed for the treatment of giant retinal tear because its recognised propensity to develop PVR. Silicone oil is favoured over long-acting gas as it ensures prolonged tamponade.

The heavy liquid/silicone oil exchange should be carried out using the wide optics of an indirect viewing system. Silicone is injected via the infusion cannula and the endo-illumination probe and a flute needle are inserted into the other two ports. As the bubble of silicone oil flows into the eye, any residual aqueous should be removed before evacuation of the heavy liquid. This is done by placing the flute needle in the periphery close to the edge of the giant tear. The bubble of heavy liquid has a dome-shaped upper surface and any aqueous will be located as a meniscus of fluid in the periphery. Care should be taken not to tilt the eye in order to get to the periphery as the heavy liquid bubble will come to occupy the more dependent part of the eye, whilst the aqueous is displaced in the opposite direction. Complete removal of the aqueous before evacuating the heavy liquid is necessary to guard against retinal slippage. Slippage occurs when a film of aqueous is displaced posteriorly allowing the retinal edge to be lifted and subsequently folded by the advancing surface of the silicone oil bubble.

Buckling

Giant breaks which extend into inferior retina should have a gentle buckle applied to the lower part of the break as this part may not receive adequate tamponade from the silicone oil bubble. Encirclement is not necessary.

Post-Operative Management

The patient should posture for 10 to 14 days in order to ensure retina is held apposed until such time as the retinopexy has had time to develop. The silicone oil can be removed after 2–3 months. Early removal of silicone oil does not guard against the development of cataract. In patients who already show significant signs of lens opacity, the removal of silicone oil can be combined with phacoemulsification and intraocular lens implantation. Cataract removal either at the time of silicone oil removal or at a subsequent stage should include a moderate to large posterior capsulotomy as the posterior capsule tends to opacify in an eye which has had silicone oil.

Prophylaxis

There is a marked tendency for the second eye to be affected (this may be as high as 50% over a period of years) and therefore in cases of spontaneous and therefore non-traumatic breaks 360° prophylactic retinopexy should be performed to the other eye. This can be done at the time of giant break surgery, either with two or three rows of indirect laser photocoagulation or with gentle confluent cryotherapy to the pre-equatorial retina. If a diagnosis of Stickler syndrome has been established the role of prophylaxis to the second eye is more controversial.

Scleral Buckling in RRD and PVR

The aims of scleral buckling are to:

- Enhance the effect of internal tamponade agents
- Assist in the closure of retinal breaks, particularly those that are inferior and less likely to be closed by tamponade
- Provide a broad-based support to the vitreous base in cases of anterior PVR.

Scleral buckling can enhance the effect of internal tamponade agents. No tamponade agent be it gas or silicone oil can be expected to provide a complete internal tamponade of all retinal areas. The various reasons for this were discussed in Chap. 7, the main one being that it is difficult to achieve a total tamponade of a near-spherical cavity. Scleral buckling mounts breaks on an indent to ensure closure of the breaks by the tamponade agent. If breaks are inferior they should be supported on relatively high buckles, radial if single or circumferential if multiple. More usually there will be associated anterior PVR and a broad buckle is used to support the vitreous base combined with an encircling procedure to ensure permanence (a 40 band overlying a 287 or 279 tyre is suitable).

Relieving Retinotomies and Retinectomies

Indications

Relieving retinal incisions and retinectomy should be used after attempted removal of all epiretinal membranes when:

- When the retina cannot be reattached due to residual traction
- Irreversible shortening is present even when retinal membranes have been removed.

If it is judged that the degree of PVR (particularly anterior PVR) is so severe that it is not possible to relieve traction upon the retina and to close retinal breaks with dissection and buckling or if after removal of ERM, retina is incapable of reattachment due to shortening, then further steps must be taken

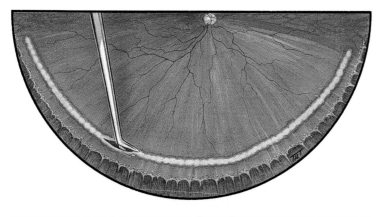

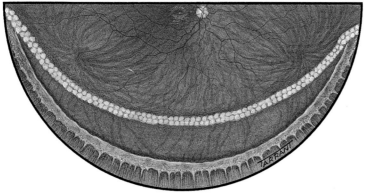

Fig. 16.5. After membrane peel retinotomy is performed to relieve residual traction. Endo-laser photocoagulation seals the posterior edge of the break.

to achieve reattachment. A retinotomy is usually a circumferential incision of the retina parallel to the ora serrata extending for a greater or lesser part of the 360° (Fig. 16.5). Isolated anterior retina is removed (retinectomy) to reduce the risk of hypotony caused by traction on the ciliary body from subsequent membranous proliferation of residual anterior retinal frill and of the risk of rubeosis due to ischaemia. The large areas of bare pigment epithelium do not appear to be deleterious.

Surgical Sequence

This involves:

- Testing the relieve of traction with heavy liquid and deciding where to make the incision and to what extent

- Removing the heavy liquids and applying endo-diathermy
- Retinotomy and retinectomy
- Further assessment of the relief of traction by re-introducing heavy liquid injection
- Endo-laser
- Inferior iridectomy
- Fluid/air exchange
- Injection of tamponade agent.

Deciding Where and How Much

If a retinotomy is to be performed it is done so after complete dissection of epiretinal membrane in the posterior retina. A partial fill with heavy liquid re-apposes posterior retina to the pigment epithelium and also gives some idea of the extent of anterior traction allowing an estimation of how extensive or posterior a retinotomy needs to be. For the majority of cases, the unrelieved traction is concentrated at the vitreous base where the basal gel and epiretinal membranes are most adherent to the underlying retina. The usual place for the retinotomy is, therefore, at the posterior border of the vitreous base. However, if anterior traction systems are extensive, then a more posterior incision needs to be made (particularly likely in re-operations)

Circumferential Extent

Smaller retinotomies have a tendency to fail due to re-proliferation at the ends of the relieving retinal incisions. Retinotomies should not be less than 180° unless the PVR is extremely localised (e.g. local proliferation associated with a perforation site).

Removal of the Heavy Liquid and Endo-Diathermy

Having noted where the retinal incision is going to be made, the heavy liquid is removed. A row of diathermy is applied to prepare the retina for retinotomy.

Retinotomy and Retinectomy

Retinotomy can be made using intraocular scissors or using a vitrectomy probe. Cutting with scissors is more controlled, but cutting with the vitrectomy probe using low suction can also be precise and efficient. Note that the retinotomy is usually made after most if not all the heavy liquid has been previously removed. Otherwise, the heavy liquid approximates the retina to the retinal pigment epithelium making it difficult to insinuate the blade of the scissors to cut the retina without the risk of touching and damaging the underlying retinal pigment epithelium and also of risking choroidal touch and haemorrhage. After retinotomy the isolated retina and attached vitreous gel are removed up to the ora serrata using deep indentation.

Further Testing of Traction Relief by Re-injection of Heavy Liquid

After the retinotomy and retinectomy the heavy liquid is re-introduced. If the judgement on traction relief and siting of the retinotomy was correct, the retina should be totally re-apposed. If in spite of retinotomy the posterior retinal edge is still somewhat tense this tension is relieved by the use of radial incisions. This is done after heavy liquid has been partially removed and further membrane peeling and retinal incisions made until complete retinal re-apposition with heavy liquid has been achieved.

Endo-Laser

Endo-laser is carried out to the cut edge of the retina. If a retinotomy is less than 360° in extent, it is important to apply endo-laser to cover the pre-equatorial retina in the uncut clock hours up to the ora serrata to seal the extremities.

Fluid/Air Exchange

A fluid/air exchange is then carried out. Care should be taken at this stage to avoid slippage. At the end of the exchange, the eye is air filled and inflated to a preset pressure. It is worthwhile waiting 5 minutes and fluting the last drop of fluid from the eye before injecting silicone oil. This duration of time is needed for the air to compress and completely displace any aqueous from any residual gel in the vitreous base. This manoeuvre allows a maximum silicone oil fill which will be achieved by infusing silicone oil either via the infusion cannula (if 1000 cs oil is used) or via a short cannula through one of the upper two sclerotomies (if 5000 cs oil is used).

Alternatively, a direct heavy liquid/silicone oil exchange can be carried out. By virtue of their surface energies silicone oil preferentially forms an interface with heavy liquid. Paradoxically, any residual vitreous fluid (aqueous) will be located above the incoming silicone oil bubble even though silicone has a lower specific gravity than aqueous. Posterior displacement of aqueous does not occur so readily and slippage is less likely to occur. When large retinotomies are used scleral buckles are unnecessary.

Avoiding slippage
• Wide-angle optics are essential for this stage of the procedure
• Keep the eye in the primary position
• The vitreous cavity should be filled as full as possible with heavy liquids
• When the air or silicone oil is infused the flute needle should be directed at the interface of the heavy liquid anteriorly and peripherally to aspirate any residual aqueous
• Rotating the eye to visualise this interface will cause the aqueous to flow away from view as the heavy liquids gravitates to occupy the more dependent part of the vitreous cavity
• Elimination of any residual aqueous from the vitreous cavity will avoid slippage
• Elimination of any residual aqueous from the vitreous cavity will avoid slippage

Complications of Retinotomy

Per-operative

Subretinal Heavy Liquid

If a retinotomy is fashioned too anteriorly and there is unrelieved traction posterior to the cut edge, heavy liquid will enter the subretinal space.

Action

When this complication happens, all the heavy liquid needs to be removed and further dissection should be undertaken to relieve posterior traction. This complication should be prevented by proper testing of the extent of traction relief with heavy liquid before making the retinotomy.

Haemorrhage

If bleeding is encountered during retinotomy, the infusion pressure should be raised and further

diathermy applied. The fundal view can be lost quickly if the bleeding is profuse. Haemorrhage from the retinal edge collects both in the pre-retinal and the subretinal compartments and unless evacuated quickly will clot, making subsequent removal more difficult. Any residual blood clots on the surface of the retina or the retinal pigment epithelium will form scaffolding for subsequent proliferation and membrane formation. Choroidal haemorrhage may occur if scissors scrape pigment epithelium.

Action

Raise the bottle, cease further retinotomy and apply further endo-diathermy. An aspirating diathermy probe is useful for the purpose as it provides the facility to aspirate, back flush and diathermize in a single 20-gauge instrument.

Post-operative

In addition to the complications of vitrectomy, of gas or oil tamponade, there are complications specific to retinotomy and retinectomy and these are:

• Re-detachment
• Post-operative hypotony
• Blockage of inferior iridectomy.

If re-detachment following retinotomy occurs, it may be due to elevation of the cut edge, or from a posterior retinal break. The detachment is often shallow but readily detected by biomicroscopy. Posterior retinal breaks can be dealt with by oil removal and further membrane peel and endo-laser. If the offending break is from the edge of the retinectomy, and the edge is noted to be thickened and fibrotic, then further retinotomies need to be fashioned. Such incisions are made circumferentially and parallel to the original retinotomy edge. If in spite of re-detachment the PVR process responsible for the detachment is only localised, at the time of re-operation silicone oil may be removed and replaced, this time with gas tamponade and further retinopexy. This will obviate silicone oil removal at a later date.

A low intraocular pressure is the usual sequel to retinectomy. This may be due to increased uveoscleral outflow of aqueous. Proliferation around the anterior frill of retina and vitreous base may interfere with aqueous production of the ciliary processes.

Rationale of Long-Acting Tamponade

After retinal traction has been relieved the object of long-acting tamponade (weeks or months) is to maintain break closure and retinal reattachment and thus abolish the stimulus for ERM production.

Choice of Long-Acting Internal Tamponade Agents

The choice between long-acting gas (e.g. C3F8) and oil is dictated by the surgeon's individual experience. The following points need to be considered:

- Theoretically gas provides a better arc of contact than oil for a given fill
- Gas top-up may be necessary
- The use of silicone oil leads to early visual rehabilitation and this is much appreciated in patients who may already have had several procedures
- Oil has to be removed whenever possible at a later date
- Long-term complications of silicone oil are probably greater than those of gas

Theoretically, gas gives a larger arc of retinal contact than silicone oil for the same volume of fill. If gas is used, then post-operative 'top-up' injections are necessary to ensure an adequate volume of tamponade for a sufficiently long period. The action of silicone oil is permanent while it is in the eye but it is difficult to ensure a good fill.

The refractive index of oil is closer to that of ocular media than gas and therefore gives rise to early visual rehabilitation. In the phakic or pseudophakic eye the refraction shifts markedly in the hypermetropic direction (usually about 5 or 6 dioptres). Spectacle correction of this error is usually unsatisfactory due to anisometropia and contact lens wear is seldom satisfactory. Ideally,

silicone oil should be removed in all cases with the object of improving vision (by removing the refractive error and sometimes annoying variations of vision from which these patients suffer) and also to avoid complications from its long-term use (particularly glaucoma). However, if the patient is exhausted by multiple procedures and there is reasonable vision in the other eye, then the long retention of silicone may be preferable. The removal of silicone oil will not always result in significant visual improvement but is sometimes disastrously complicated by re-detachment of the retina. No attempt at removal of silicone should be made if there are observed to be unresolved or recurrent tractional retinal systems.

The timing of silicone oil removal is arbitrary. Early removal, say within 6 weeks, cannot be relied on to prevent progression of cataract formation. However, the incidence of glaucoma increases, the longer the oil is left in situ. Once glaucoma has developed, removal of oil does not render the eye normotensive but facilitates the management of a raised pressure.

Prolonged silicone oil tamponade may be associated with peri-oil fibrosis and macular pucker. A reasonable compromise between the need for prolonged tamponade and inactivation of the PVR process and the wish to avoid long-term complications is to remove silicone oil 3–6 months after surgery. This can be combined with phacoemulsification of any cataract that has formed and also further dissection of simple epiretinal membranes (e.g. causing macular pucker).

Re-detachment

Re-detachment of the retina occurs as a result of missed or unclosed breaks and recurrent PVR (Fig. 16.6). It is rare for new breaks to form. In a silicone-filled eye the re-detachment is almost invariably inferior but in spite of the presence of the silicone oil bubble the contour is usually convex towards the vitreous cavity. This indicates the presence of an open retinal break. Less frequently, a traction-like detachment with a border that is concave towards the vitreous cavity will appear. This is not associated with an open retinal break and is not usually progressive.

At re-operation, simple surgery with scleral buckling to close a retinal break is not usually adequate.

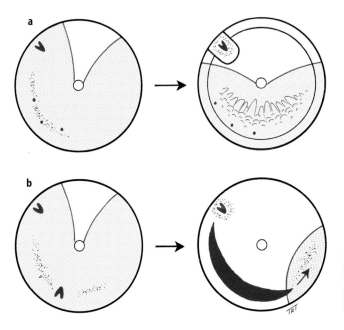

Fig. 16.6. a Local and encircling buckle and PPV has failed to seal a break and extensive inferior PVR has developed; **b** a retinotomy has been performed to deal with extensive inferior PVR. However, one edge of the retinotomy has reopened due to reproliferation of epiretinal membrane and localised redetachment has occurred. The retinotomy should have been bigger.

A further retinotomy and retinectomy is usually required to remove recurrent PVR.

In the eye that already contains silicone oil there is usually no urgency for re-operation and this will allow time for the patient to recover before the rigours of further surgery.

> Will further surgery be of benefit to your patient?

When Not to Operate

Surgical enthusiasm must be tempered by good judgement in deciding on when and when not to advise surgery for advanced PVR. The age of the patient, the state of the other eye, the general health and the visual needs and demands of the individual patient together with the economics of prolonged repeated surgery are all factors that have to be considered when deciding to pursue a complex surgical option. The likely long-term benefits must be carefully assessed and will vary from one patient to another. A series of operations on a relatively young patient to restore at least some vision may be acceptable (unless the patient is severely ill, e.g. in CMV retinitis) but will rarely be so in an elderly patient (say over the age of 80) in whom there is normal vision in the healthy other eye.

Some patients, very reluctant to let an eye go blind, will be enthusiastic for more surgery while others will be adamant in declining further procedures. However, the majority of patients will be dependent on the surgeon to advise them on whether or not further surgery should be performed. In these complex cases the decision is made jointly with the patient after a full explanation of the risks and expectations. This explanation is not easy as the surgical outcome is often unpredictable, both anatomically and visually. Also, there is uncertainty about the patients reaction to any improvement. Thus a small increase in vision may be greeted with enthusiasm by some (for example increase in field may help driving a motor car) while others are less happy, even complaining that the blurred vision in the operated eye has become more obvious than pre-operatively and interferes with the other eye.

In general, successful surgery will improve field of vision, but central vision is likely to remain poor although any pre-operative metamorphopsia may be improved. Patient and surgeon have to consider whether these potential gains are worthwhile.

Results

Even in advanced cases anatomical reattachment can be achieved in approximately 75% of cases.

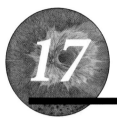

17 Pars Plana Vitrectomy: Post-operative Management and Complications

PPV Using Gas

The degree of post-operative disturbance of the eye will reflect the complexity of the procedure. Eyes that have been treated without scleral buckling will be remarkably quiet. The patient will experience little more than discomfort. This discomfort will be much increased if extensive buckling procedures have been performed, particularly in eyes that have had previous surgery.

General Advice

Those patients who had good vision prior to surgery should be warned that gas within the vitreous cavity severely limits vision. This warning will avoid alarm in the immediate post-operative period and patients are warned that vision will not start to improve until the lower meniscus of the gas bubble has reached the midline allowing macular vision. This will usually take 1–2 weeks from the time of surgery. After this time vision should rapidly improve if the retina is securely reattached. The gas bubble is perceived as a mobile black shadow and a warning should be given that it may break up into one or more bubbles as its size diminishes. If this is to happen it usually does so a day or two before complete absorption.

Posture

Posturing in the post-operative period is extremely important with the twin objectives of achieving break tamponade and also avoiding contact of the gas bubble with the posterior lens capsule in the phakic eye to prevent cataract. Posture commences as soon as possible after surgery (the same day) and is arranged so that the break is in the superior position. This position must be achieved for as much of the day as possible and the sleeping position must also be adapted to achieve this effect. If breaks are separated by a wide arc of retina (about 140°) then post-operative tamponade may not be relied upon to close both sets of breaks. In these cases it is probably wiser to have buckled the smaller of the breaks and to concentrate the head position to tamponade the more complex break. Although the bubble remains in the eye for a variable length of time 10 days appears to be completely adequate for adhesion and sealing of a break in an eye uncomplicated by significant PVR.

Post-operative Activity

During this time much activity is not usually possible and flying is contraindicated because of bubble expansion during the unpressurised phase of aircraft ascent (causing pain, glaucoma, and central retinal artery occlusion) and hypotony on descent (risking intraocular haemorrhage). After absorption of the gas bubble the management of patients is exactly the same as that following conventional retinal detachment surgery.

Complications

PPV risks the same complications as those following conventional retinal detachment procedures but if the PPV procedure has not involved the use of scleral buckles then it has the outstanding advantage that all post-operative complications of buckles are avoided (diplopia, enophthalmos, explant infection, or anterior segment ischaemia).

Specific post-operative anterior segment complications of gas tamponade procedures are:

- Early feather-like subcapsular lens opacities are often seen in the phakic eye on the first day or two after surgery (Fig. 17.1). This change is reversible by correct posturing to prevent gas bubble contact with the posterior lens capsule (if more than one third of the posterior lens capsule is in contact with the bubble then these opacities will appear).
- Glaucoma. Transient open angle glaucoma is quite common. Medical treatment in the form of

local timolol or systemic acetazolamide is all that is necessary to control pressure which may persist for a week or two following surgery.

- In pseudophakic eyes the intraocular lens may be found to have become partially dislocated or pupil capture may have occurred. These changes are usually caused by forward movement of the lens-iris diaphragm associated with gas in the posterior segment. It is uncommon for any specific surgical treatment to be necessary but if severely displaced the intraocular lens may need re-positioning.
- Late lens opacity. Progressive nuclear sclerosis is the most important late complication of PPV in the phakic eye (see Chap. 14). These lens opacities cause increasing lenticular myopia about which the patient must be warned as initial excellent vision is progressively reduced as the lens opacity develops. Nuclear sclerosis is almost inevitable in patients over the age of 50 but may not develop in younger patients. Extracapsular lens extraction with intraocular lens implantation is carried out when visual disturbance is marked and this can be done with no fear of re-detachment of the retina. The occurrence of these lens opacities is the reason why it is right to try to reattach the retina with conventional external buckling techniques if this is possible even though on some occasions conventional buckling may be technically more difficult and time-consuming than simple PPV.

Posterior Segment

Re-detachment of the retina is by far the most important 'complication' (see Chap. 15).

PPV Using Silicone Oil: Post-Operative Management and Complications

Posture

The objective of silicone oil tamponade is to achieve as total a fill as possible. Practically, this is never achieved (see Chap. 8). Post-operatively, residual vitreous will be compressed by the oil creating

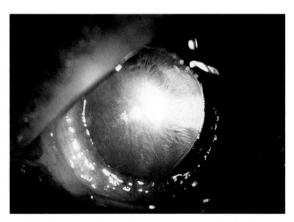

Fig. 17.1. Feathery gas lens opacities seen in the immediate post-operative period.

under-fill. If no explants were used and the silicone oil is expected to tamponade the inferior fundus (e.g. a giant retinal tear extending below the horizontal or a 360° retinectomy), patients need to posture appropriately (on their sides or head down) for the usual 7–10 days in order to increase the effectiveness of the tamponade. If all inferior breaks are mounted on explants, there is no need to posture.

Complications

The complications associated with PPV and silicone oil are:

- Raised intraocular pressure
- Refractive change
- Cataract formation
- Emulsification of oil
- Silicone oil keratopathy
- Peri-oil fibrosis
- Re-detachment of the retina

Other complications are those related to retinal detachment, either as a result of failure of the surgical operation to reattach the retina or following silicone oil removal.

Raised Intraocular Pressure in the Early Post-operative Period

- Aphakic eyes
- Phakic and pseudophakic eyes.

In the aphakic eye, raised intraocular pressure can occur in the early post-operative period as a result of pupil block glaucoma. It is not unusual for the intraocular pressure to rise above 50 mmHg. The eye becomes painful although corneal oedema may be absent. Pupil block glaucoma can be prevented by the use of an inferior peripheral iridectomy. Silicone oil has a lower specific gravity than that of aqueous (0.97), and tends to occupy the upper part of the vitreous cavity; thus to allow communication between the anterior and posterior chambers the peripheral iridectomy needs to be in the six o'clock position. Blockage of the peripheral iridectomy by

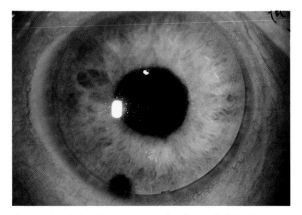

Fig. 17.2. An inferior iridectomy is present but silicone oil is filling the anterior chamber.

inflammatory debris and organised tissue, may be exacerbated by the retention of capsular remnants. Adequate control of uveitis is therefore important and this involves pre-operative treatment with systemic non-steroidal anti-inflammatory agents, subconjunctival steroid at the end of surgery and intensive post-operative topical steroid. Patients are instructed to posture with their heads tilted forward which will allow aqueous to flow from the posterior segment into the anterior chamber. This is particularly important if the anterior chamber becomes partially filled with silicone during oil injection at surgery. With posture, the smaller bubble of silicone oil in the anterior chamber will move into the large one in the vitreous cavity (this occurs naturally in order to achieve a lower surface energy) provided a patent channel is available for aqueous to move in the other direction to reform the anterior chamber (Fig. 17.2).

Pupil block can be recognised by the presence of oil in the anterior chamber. The signs include:

- A widely dilated pupil
- An exudative membrane over the iridectomy
- Lack of an oil/aqueous interface in the pupillary plane

Prevention of pupil blockage

- By performing a peripheral iridectomy.
- By early post-operative posturing.
- By adequate suppression of inflammation

- Absence of flare in the anterior chamber because the anterior chamber is filled with oil
- Reflections of the oil in the iris crypts

In the phakic or pseudophakic eye, early raised intraocular pressure can arise from true overfill. The physical signs are:

1. Herniation of oil between the pupil and lens
2. Shallowing of the anterior chamber.

This can best be treated by prevention:

- Do not leave the eye at a high intraocular pressure at the end of the operation
- Do not close sclerotomies before buckles are secured after oil injection. This is particularly the case when encircling elements are used as they can stretch and store up tension.

In an eye without silicone oil high pressure leads to an increase in aqueous outflow which lowers and normalises the intraocular pressure. However, in an eye filled with oil, the only aqueous available is that in the anterior chamber and high intraocular pressure will lead to shallowing of the anterior chamber. If the eye was left hard at the end of surgery, there may not be sufficient aqueous to flow out of the eye to normalise the intraocular pressure post-operatively. Similarly, the tension stored by a tight encirclement has the effect of increasing intraocular pressure post-operatively which may or may not be compensated for by aqueous outflow.

A true overfill can sometimes be managed by aspiration of some of the silicone oil via the pars plana. Where the oil is herniating between the pupil and the lens, this film of oil is trapped. Simple aspiration of the oil from the posterior segment will not relieve this pupil block, which will only be achieved by complete removal of oil from the eye. In the aphakic eye, overfill may be relieved by paracentesis.

> Silicone-filled eyes need regular follow-up indefinitely

Raised Intraocular Pressure in the Late Post-operative Period

Causes include:

- Emulsification of silicone
- Pre-existing glaucoma
- Steroid-induced glaucoma
- Uveitis.

On gonioscopy the angle is seen to be opened and small droplets may be seen superiorly.

Most patients following vitrectomy are treated with several weeks of topical steroid. Steroid-induced glaucoma is a diagnosis of exclusion.

Pre-existing glaucoma may be a cause of rise of intraocular pressure following reattachment of a detached retina. Raised intraocular pressure may not be obvious pre-operatively due to the increase uveo-scleral outflow afforded by the retinal detachment. Reattachment surgery reduces this outflow facility and restores the eye to its pre-operative status.

Uveitis associated with complex vitrectomy may cause secondary glaucoma. Vitrectomy causes a breakdown of the blood ocular barrier and the surgical trauma induced by manipulation of the iris or incision of the retina further promotes an inflammatory response, a response that is enhanced if there has been intraocular haemorrhage. Anti-inflammatory treatment should be directed at the exudative as well as the cellular response to the surgery. Chronic uveitis should be distinguished by emulsification of silicone oil. Fine droplets of silicone oil can mimic cells in the anterior chamber.

Management

Mild glaucoma can be managed with topical medical treatment. Persistently high intraocular pressure is a most serious complication. Nothing is more disappointing to perform one or more vitreo-retinal procedures on a patient resulting in reattachment to have the benefits of surgery removed by sight loss from glaucoma. The treatment of silicone oil glaucoma usually requires silicone oil removal combined with post-operative medical treatment. Removal of the silicone oil alone does not usually solve the glaucoma and conventional drainage surgery such trabeculectomy has little part to play. Persistently high intraocular pressure may require more aggressive treatment such as Molteno tube drainage and sometimes cyclo-ablation (the most popular method at the moment is cyclodiode laser treatment). These procedures are not without risk (drainage surgery may be complicated by suprachoroidal haemorrhage), inadequate treatment gives rise to recurrence of glaucoma and excessive treatment can lead to hypotony and phthisis. Retinal surgeons are well advised to request advice from their glaucoma colleagues early in the management of raised intraocular pressure rather then delay such advice until virtually all sight has been lost!

Cataract

All patients undergoing vitrectomy with silicone oil tamponade should be warned of this occurrence before surgery. These cataracts tend to come on within the first year after surgery leading to progressive diminution of central vision, a change that is often accompanied by increasing lenticular myopia. In the late stages, dense cataract can progress quickly to hypermaturity with swelling of the lens and shallowing of the anterior chamber. The lens may not become cataractous in young patients.

Treatment

There is controversy as to the best means of treating silicone oil cataract.

The options include:

- Cataract extraction alone, leaving the oil in situ
- Cataract extraction combined with oil removal
- Cataract extraction, oil removal and insertion of intraocular lens

The method of choice is phacoemulsification, which has superseded the earlier methods of intracapsular and standard extracapsular extractions. Extraction may be combined with silicone oil removal and insertion of intraocular lens provided it is judged that the posterior segment is stable (this is much more likely to be confidently predicted when silicone has been used for posterior proliferative con-

ditions such as in diabetes, rather than for anterior PVR). An anterior chamber infusion is used (obviating the need for pars plana perforation) and a peroperative capsulotomy provides access to the posterior segment for oil removal. Posterior chamber intraocular lens implants can be inserted in the capsular bag or in the sulcus supported by the anterior capsule. If an intraocular lens implant is used, care should be exercised to avoid contact of the intraocular lens with the silicone oil. Intraocular lenses made of polymethylmethacrylate, hydrogel or silicone material all have an affinity for silicone and oil droplets can become permanently adherent to the lens surface.

In general, when the retinal problem has been very complex (e.g. the management of extensive PVR) then the intraocular lens option is unlikely to be useful, particularly if there is reasonable vision in the other eye. Lens implantation should not be used if there is residual instablility of the posterior segment in the form of residual detachment or obvious recurrence of epiretinal membranes as the presence of an intraocular lens will only complicate the management of subsequent posterior segment surgery. If an intraocular lens is not used and silicone oil is left in situ as a permanent tamponade, then an inferior iridectomy to avoid pupil block should be made..

The precise timing of cataract surgery should be considered in relation to the desired duration of silicone oil tamponade. If the silicone oil is intended to stay in an eye for 6 months or more then a combined cataract and oil removal procedure is both economical and reasonable.

If silicone oil has already been removed from an eye and the retina has remained attached then the subsequent cataract formation can be managed in the usual way.

Emulsification of Silicone Oil

Emulsification is an invariable complication of the use of silicone oil. It is important to appreciate that emulsification can be subclinical. The dimension of emulsified droplets can be smaller than the wavelength of light and cannot be discerned by slit-lamp biomicroscopy. Larger droplets are seen as 'cells' in the anterior chamber and can be mistaken for iritis. Progressive accumulation of these droplets in the

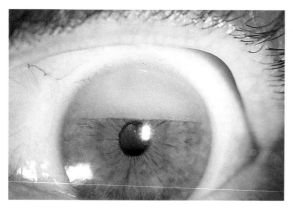

Fig. 17.3. Emulsification of silicone oil in the anterior chamber.

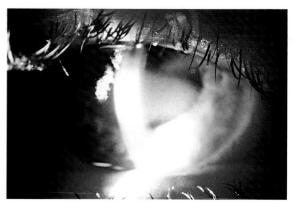

Fig. 17.4. Band-shaped keratopathy associated with silicone oil.

upper part of the anterior chamber can form a fluid level and is sometimes refer to as an inverse hypopyon (Fig. 17.3). The occurrence is rare with highly purified high viscosity (5000 cs upwards) silicone oil.

The lower the viscosity of silicone oil the greater is the likelihood of emulsification. The viscosity is determined by the molecular weight of the siloxane molecules. Highly purified oils have a more homogenous component of a single molecular weight. More importantly it should have less of the lower molecular weight siloxane and a lower tendency to emulsify. If the plan is to use silicone oil for prolonged internal tamponade, then 5000 cS highly purified silicone oil is preferred.

Droplets in the anterior chamber can obscure vision and fundal view, especially when the patient is supine. Progressive accumulation of emulsified droplets can only be effectively treated by removal of silicone oil from the vitreous cavity combined with a paracentesis and a washout of the anterior chamber. At the time of removal of the oil bubble from the vitreous cavity emulsified droplets can be adherent to the surface of the ciliary processes, retina and iris. One or more washout procedures may be needed to clear the eye of these droplets.

cification in the degenerative cornea. Eventually, peripheral corneal neovascularisation and complete corneal opacification occur.

Prevention

Although it may be necessary in some cases to remove the crystalline lens to deal with PVR preserving the lens when possible greatly reduces the risk of silicone oil keratopathy.

Treatment

Photokeratectomy (with excimer laser) can be very effective in achieving symptomatic relief when calcific plaques ulcerate causing pain and inflammation. If the eye still has visual potential the silicone oil should be removed if possible; however, this will sometimes result in decompensation of the cornea and corneal grafting may be necessary.

Oil Keratopathy

Keratopathy occurs when the anterior chamber is filled with silicone oil. The early appearance is that of horizontal band of opacity within the cornea (Fig. 17.4). Late keratopathy shows ectopic cal-

Signs of A.C. oil
• High reflexes from iris crypts
• Dilated pupils
• Absence of flare

Peri-oil Fibrosis

Proliferation of membrane may continue in cases of aggressive PVR and these membranes may form at the pre-retinal surface behind the silicone oil. The space between the oil and the retina (mainly the inferior retina where there is no contact between oil and retinal surface) consists of aqueous which contains water soluble factors active in promoting the PVR process. These membranes, often widely infiltrated with emulsified oil, are of a thick porridge-like consistency and quite adherent to the retina.

Detachment of The Retina

Detachment of the retina may occur either when silicone oil is still within the eye or as a complication following its removal. The re-detachment of the retina subsequent to PPV and the injection of silicone oil is usually due to a combination of open breaks and residual and unrelieved tangential traction upon them, with or without progression of tractional systems elsewhere on the retina. The presence of silicone oil within the eye usually confines re-detachment to the inferior retina. Sometimes breaks are sealed and tractional retinal detachment alone is present. In either situation simple removal of silicone oil will invariably result in more extensive retinal re-detachment. Although surgery involving buckling and membrane peeling may be enough to achieve retinal reattachment, it is more likely that retinotomy and retinectomy will be required. Silicone oil should be retained in the eye until its removal is deemed safe.

In spite of apparently securely reattached retina with no sign of recurrence of peri-retinal membrane or of open breaks, removal of silicone oil will sometime result in recurrence of retinal detachment. This re-detachment usually occurs within a week or two of the removal of silicone and is a very disappointing event for both patient and surgeon. It is usually caused by the reopening of retinal breaks by unrecognised traction upon them from peri-retinal membranes or from breaks inadequately treated with retinopexy. This occurrence is best prevented by ensuring adequate relief of traction at the time of initial surgery. If re-detachment does occur, re-operation will be necessary. This will usually involve replacement of silicone combined with relief of the tractional systems and sealing of the retinal breaks.

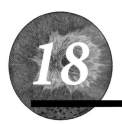

18 Pars Plana Vitrectomy for Proliferative Diabetic Retinopathy

Vitrectomy for Diabetic Retinopathy

A patient needing vitreo-retinal surgery does so as a complication of the proliferative process (PDR). This results from either failure to detect proliferative retinopathy in time for laser photocoagulation to be effective (if there is no ophthalmic screening service in position all those in charge of diabetics must be adequately skilled in ophthalmoscopy, e.g. general practitioners and diabetologists) or failure of photocoagulation to control the process. The latter failure may be due either to non-co-operation, or to inadequate photocoagulation. It is rare for an eye that has been adequately treated with full photocoagulation to come to vitreo-retinal surgery. The majority of patients developing proliferative diabetic retinopathy are insulin dependent and will have had diabetes for many years. The appearance of PDR and other serious diabetic complications such as renal failure is less frequent in those who have had good diabetic control (as measured by blood sugar levels) than those whose control has been poor.

Surgical Pathology of PDR

Pathogenesis

- Capillary non-perfusion
- New vessel formation
- Vitreous detachment
- Haemorrhage, retro-hyaloid and intra-gel
- Fibrous proliferation
- Tractional retinal detachment (TRD: also tractional schisis)
- Rhegmatogenous and traction retinal detachment.

The basic change in the retinal circulation is that of capillary non-perfusion with resultant retinal ischaemia. Locally elaborated growth factors lead to new vessel formation. This new vessel formation is usually confined to the retinal circulation (proliferative retinopathy) but sometimes the anterior segment is affected (rubeosis iridis). New vessels usually arise from arterio-venous crossings. This new vessel formation is mainly situated in the vessels at the posterior pole, either at the disc itself or from the vessels of the major arcades. New vessels may occur as peripheral at the equatorial retina. The vessels grow initially within the plane of the retina and eventually grow forward from it into the vitreous cortex. PDR encourages posterior vitreous detachment. When vitreous traction is exerted upon them by the detaching posterior hyaloid the new vessels may bleed producing vitreous haemorrhage. Infiltration by fibrotic tissue results in the conversion of a purely vascular complex to a fibrovascular one (retinitis proliferans). This system contracts and results in traction at its points of attachment to the retina (Fig. 18.1).

The progression of PDR is related to the attachments of the vitreous gel. Unusually, if there is a complete posterior vitreous detachment the posterior segment can be spared from neovascularisation while rubeosis iridis develops in the anterior segment. If new vessels develop behind a detached gel they tend to do so either as small innocuous fibrovascular clumps or as flat disc vessels. Thus, the vitreous gel provides a collagen scaffolding upon which new vessels may proliferate. If haemorrhages occur they may be intra-gel or retro-hyaloid. If retro-hyaloid the blood collections in a partially detached gel may have a fluid level and take on a semi-lunar shape.

Effect of Static Traction Upon the Retina

In addition to vitreous haemorrhage, contraction of the posterior hyaloid causing static traction upon the retina can result in a variety of clinical appearances; these are:

- Avulsed loops of blood vessels
- Intraretinal separation: traction retinoschisis
- Retinal detachment: TRD
- Retinal holes: combined TRD and RRD.

Avulsed loops of blood vessels (usually retinal veins) are common and may be confused with new blood vessel, and care is needed when excising membranes during vitrectomy as these loops may be divided by mistake. Static traction can produce intraretinal separation (traction retinoschisis). Diaphanous areas within the schisis are sometime mistaken for retinal breaks. TRD is produced by fibrovascular proliferative areas and these areas of

detachment are usually sited around the optic disc and vascular arcades.

Tractional Systems

The various types of traction system that are common to all forms of TRD, although varying substantially in complexity from one case to another are:

- Antero-posterior traction
- Table-top detachment
- Bridging traction.

Contracture along the detached posterior vitreous face gives rise to antero-posterior traction and this is usually between the posterior border of the vitreous base and areas of retinitis proliferans (RP). Tangential traction along the surface of the retina overlies areas of RP and results in table-top detachment (Fig. 18.2). Bridging traction occurs between areas of detached retina.

The extent of posterior hyaloid separation varies quite markedly from one case to another and this, combined with the extent and site of table-top detachment, are the main features that determine the complexity of the surgical dissection. Eyes that have been treated with extensive laser photocoagulation may have very incomplete vitreous separation over the treated areas.

Retinal Breaks and Combined Rhegmatogenous and Traction Retinal Detachments

Traction upon the retina may produce full-thickness retinal breaks and they are nearly always located in close proximity to areas of fibrovascular proliferation. These breaks may, but not always, result in a rhegmatogenous element to the TRD (Fig. 18.1). Combined RRD and TRD (see Chap. 3) should be suspected when:

- The retinal detachment becomes mobile
- The retinal contour becomes convex towards the vitreous cavity and towards attached retina.
- The retinal detachment extends beyond the equator

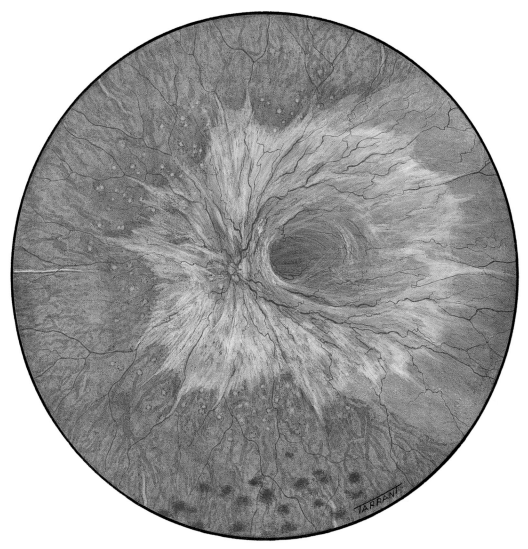

Fig. 18.1. Fundus painting to show scattered and inadequate laser photocoagulation for PDR and traction and rhegmatogenous retinal detachment.

- SRF extends through previous high-water marks associated with TRD

Rarely retinal breaks occur at the posterior border of the vitreous base, secondary to peripheral posterior vitreous detachment and RRD may spread secondarily from this break to involve central TRD. In many of these patients, extensive photocoagula-

tion has been applied and the localisation of the peripheral break may not be obvious due to the atypical distribution of SRF.

The distinction between tractional retinal detachment and tractional retinoschisis is not particularly important as treatment is not advised in either condition unless the macula is involved. High-water marks are found in relationship to static TRD, but not in retinoschisis.

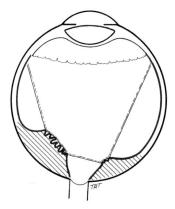

Fig. 18.2. The typical arrangement of vitreous detachment in PDR.

Surgical Assessment of Diabetic Eye Disease

Symptoms

The surgical assessment of the patient should take account of symptoms. Sudden visual loss, for example, caused by vitreous haemorrhage or detachment of the retina involving the macula is usually obvious to the patient. Gradual loss, however, is more difficult for both patient and surgeon to assess. It may be produced by a combination of factors such as cataract, vitreous haemorrhage, slow extension of TRD into the macular area or from coincidental diabetic maculopathy. The level of vision may fluctuate.

Signs

Slit-lamp biomicroscopy is used to detect the presence of rubeosis and any degree of lens opacity. In eyes with clear media, the extent of posterior vitreous detachment should be assessed pre-operatively using indirect ophthalmoscopy followed by biomicroscopy. This assessment will give an indication of the likely complexity of the dissection and outcome of the case. An example of a simple diabetic vitrectomy is that for removal of vitreous haemorrhage when the gel is detached posteriorly inserting only at the disc. A combined TRD with RRD with little vitreous detachment presents a formidable surgical challenge.

Haemorrhage

Bleeding into the vitreous cavity occurs mainly into the vitreous cortex and retro-hyaloid space (Fig. 18.3). Minor haemorrhages may clear sufficiently in a few days to allow further assessment and laser photocoagulation. Patients whose fundus is obscured should receive further investigation with B-mode ultrasound scanning to determine the extent of vitreous detachment and the position of the retina.

General Condition

An assessment should be made of the general physical condition of the patient. Many diabetic patients have multi-system problems including coronary artery disease, poor peripheral circulation and renal

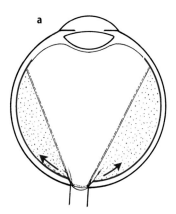
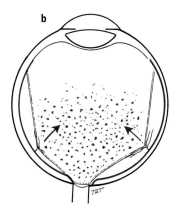

Fig. 18.3a,b. Vitreous haemorrhage in PDR.

failure. Planned surgical admissions may involve combined care with physicians, nephrologists and anaesthetists. Many patients coming to surgery are insulin dependent and insulin requirements may have to be altered over the operative period. The choice of surgery under local or general anaesthesia needs to take into account the complexity of the surgery and the risks of anaesthesia.

Aims of Surgery (PPV)

The aims of surgery are to:

- Remove vitreous opacity
- Relieve traction upon the retina
    - i. To allow TRD to settle
    - ii. To relieve distortion on the macula from vitreous traction
- Reattachment of RRD by closing and sealing full-thickness retinal breaks
- To effect metabolic control with endo-photocoagulation.

The Indications for Surgery

The indications for surgery are:

- Persistent or recurrent vitreous haemorrhage preventing adequate laser photocoagulation
- Acute pre-macular haemorrhage
- TRD involving the macula
- Macular ectopia or distortion due to distortion from contraction by neighbouring retinitis proliferans
- Rubeosis iridis with vitreous haemorrhage
- Combined rhegmatogenous and tractional detachment.

Vitreous Haemorrhage

Persistent vitreous haemorrhage usually refers to one that has been present for more than 6 months. A significant proportion of first haemorrhages will clear allowing photocoagulation to stabilise the retina. In some patients peripheral retina may be treated with laser photocoagulation delivered through the indirect ophthalmoscope particularly when central haemorrhage persists. It is desirable to apply as much photocoagulation as possible to dampen down the neovascular process before proceeding to vitrectomy. In some instances vitreous haemorrhage may be recurrent and never clear well enough for sufficient photocoagulation to achieve control. The excellent results of PPV for cases of vitreous haemorrhage of shorter duration (say 1–3 months) has to be weighted against surgical morbidity. The age of the patient, occupation and state of the other eye will all be factors in considering the need for surgery. Selecting patients with recurrent vitreous haemorrhage is difficult; if however these are repeated and adequate photocoagulation is impossible then surgery should not be unnecessarily delayed. Delay will risk extension of fibrovascular process and make eventual surgery much more difficult. Acute pre-macular haemorrhage may compromise the visual function irreversibly especially if the haemorrhage has a tense cyst-like appearance.

RRD and TRD

TRD suddenly extending to involve the macula should be regarded with the same urgency as acute RRD and should be operated upon without delay. The longer the macula has been detached by the TRD the worse will be the prognosis of the restoration of central vision following reattachment.

Combined rhegmatogenous and tractional retinal detachment is usually progressive threatening both peripheral and central vision. Vitreous surgery aims to relieve the static traction and close the offending retinal breaks. Usually this can be achieved by a combination of vitrectomy and internal tamponade and scleral buckling is seldom required.

Macular Ectopia

The vision may drop as a result of pucker or distortion of the macular as a result of traction by an adjacent area of retinitis proliferans.

Rubeosis

Eyes with active rubeosis can give rise to angle closure and irreversible rise in intraocular pressure.

This can occur rapidly. If the view is not sufficiently clear for laser treatment, early surgery offers an opportunity to avoid permanent damage to the drainage angle by the rubeotic neovascularization. If not too advanced the rubeotic process may be reversed by vitrectomy and widespread photocoagulation.

When Surgery is not Advisable

Vitrectomy is not advisable for the following conditions:

1. Extra-macular traction retinal detachments which may be stable for years
2. Longstanding retinal detachment (more than one year) involving the macula with little prospect of visual improvement even if surgically reattached
3. Complex surgical configuration and active vascular proliferation especially when the fellow eye is stable.

Extra-macular tractional detachments are often stable. If the vascular proliferation is already controlled with laser photocoagulation, these eyes can be observed. Surgery will not improve visual function if the retinal detachment has been longstanding and these patients may be observed for further signs of visual deterioration before attempting surgery.

The potential benefit of a diabetic vitrectomy needs to be weighed against the likelihood of serious complications, the most important of which are retinal breaks inducing retinal detachment, rubeosis leading to glaucoma, and cataract formation. An eye may be rendered blind and painful or phthisical.

Pre-operative Counselling

In addition to the usual information about PPV, patients undergoing PPV for PDR should receive additional counselling. They should be warned that some degree of vitreous haemorrhage is quite common in the post-operative period and this may take some weeks to clear (this information will avoid immediate disappointment after surgery). Cataract

> Rubeosis indicates that treatment is urgent

formation after vitrectomy surgery is common even in relatively young patients. Patients with TRD involving the macula should be given a guarded prognosis. Partly because the actual duration of detachment is often unclear from the history but also because of the vulnerability of macular function to damage by detachment combined with an underlying and often unpredictable degree of macular ischaemia. The patient needs to have a clear idea of the objectives of surgery and to be given a realistic appraisal of the risk of complications and visual outcome.

Surgical Techniques

Removal of Vitreous Haemorrhage

The surgical sequence is:

- Remove of central gel
- Fenestration of the posterior hyaloid face
- Aspiration of retro-hyaloid blood
- Excision of cortical gel
- Deep indentation to remove blood clots in vitreous base.

In an eye with dense vitreous haemorrhage the view of the fundus may be totally obscured. In such cases there is danger of damaging the retina particularly if retina is drawn forward by TRD.. This danger underlies the importance of pre-operative ultrasonography to help guide the surgeon in the initial phases of the dissection. The first step should be to remove the central gel haemorrhage to allow access to the posterior hyaloid face overlying attached retina. A small opening in the posterior hyaloid is made with the cutter allowing removal of the retro-hyaloid blood. This small window will allow viewing of underlying retina and will facilitate orientation and subsequent dissection. If there is no TRD, the vitreous cutter is used to enlarge this opening in the posterior vitreous face and the gel frill trimmed to the equator. Blood settling on the surface of the retina may be removed by a back flush flute needle.

Dense clots of blood are often found in the inferior vitreous base and deep indentation improves access and facilitates removal. Leaving inferior residual blood may cause:

- Post-operative haze
- Ghost-cell glaucoma.

The release of red blood cells from the gel frill tends to obscure fundal view in the early post-operative period. Red blood cells can block the trabecular meshwork and produce post-operative ghost cell glaucoma.

Removal of Vitreo-Retinal Traction

The techniques used are:

- Delamination
- En-bloc dissection
- Segmentation.

These moves are facilitated by the use of multi-function instruments.

In the presence of tractional retinal detachments the technique for vitrectomy needs to be modified. Once again, it is necessary to gain access to the retro-hyaloid compartment early in the operative procedure. Instruments are then inserted underneath the intact hyaloid and blunt dissection is carried out to gently lift the fibrovascular membranes from the retina. The purpose of the blunt dissection is to create a tissue plane for dissection. Fibrovascular membranes are usually attached to

the retina by feeder blood vessels. The dissection of vascular membranes is entirely different from that used for non-vascularized membranes of PVR. No attempt should be made to 'peel' these membranes otherwise avulsion of these feeder vessels from retinal vessels will give rise to bleeding which is difficult to control. Any traction on the retina either deliberate in the form of peeling or inadvertent will tend to produce breaks in the thin underlying diabetic retina. Once the correct tissue plane is identified by blunt dissection, angled scissors are used to divide these feeder vessels. The process of removal of the fibrovascular membranes along with the posterior hyaloid is referred to as delamination (Fig. 18.4). The posterior vitreous face should be kept intact as this will provide a degree of anterior posterior traction on the membranes which is helpful to dissection.

PDR surgery
Complexity depends on the extent of the PVD

Occasionally, there are areas of firm adhesions between a fibrovascular membrane and the detached retina. Traction on the membranes simply causes the retina to become more elevated and sharp dissection may run the risk of forming iatrogenic retinal breaks. In these instances it is more expedient to cut around the membrane leaving this an island of tissue. The membrane may then be divided into segments using vertical scissors in order to relieve the tangential traction upon the surface of the retina. The degree of complexity of delamination is largely determined by the area and strength of adhesion between the fibrovascular membrane and the underlying retina. If connections are very small then the dissection is rapid with little risk of complication such as haemorrhage or retinal break formation. If on the other hand, the connection is extensive then the dissection will be laborious and time consuming with a higher risk of complications. It is not usually advisable to completely remove fronds of neovascular tissue from the optic disc. These fronds will have to be shortened leaving a small residual stub of tissue. Occasionally multi-function probes such as illuminated picks or those combining an aspiration cannula with a

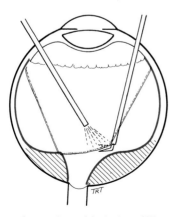

Fig. 18.4. Scissor delamination at PPV.

light pipe may be useful. They allow membranes to be purchased with one instrument and cut with another thus facilitating segmentation and delamination.

Haemostasis and Endo-diathermy

Bleeding can arise during membrane dissection. Dividing feeder vessels to the membrane often causes surprising little amount of haemorrhage even when the vessels are quite large. However when feeder vessels are avulsed, they tear away from the retinal venules from which they arise. These retinal bleeding points are difficult to control and removal of clotted blood can be awkward. Other sources of bleeding may be vascular loops that can be accidentally mistaken for new vessels and from the cut edge of neovascular fronds which have been shortened on the disc. Endo-diathermy is often ineffective and if heavy runs the risk of creating breaks. The infusion bottle is raised to encourage haemostasis.

Laser Photocoagulation

Per-operative laser photocoagulation is invariably performed for all cases of proliferative diabetic retinopathy which come to vitrectomy and usually involves one or more of the following approaches:

1. Treatment of post-equatorial retina (with straight or curved endo-laser probes)
2. Treatment of pre-equatorial retina with deep indentation.
3. Treatment of coincidental diabetic maculopathy
4. Per-operative treatment of retinal breaks.

Once the media is cleared, and fibrovascular membranes removed, it is possible to treat the retina with endo-laser photocoagulation. Endo-laser can be used to fill in gaps in previous photocoagulation and if the vascular proliferation is very active, over-treatment of previously photocoagulated retina can be performed. Deep indentation allows treatment of pre-equatorial retina. This can be carried as a bimanual technique using the coaxial illumination of the operating microscope with the laser probe held in one hand and a scleral indentor in the other. (Alternatively, a combined endo-illumination and laser probe is available and convenient to use). A

curved laser probe can ensure a more even uptake of laser energy by directing the beam perpendicular to the retinal surface. Occasionally, it is convenient to deliver the laser via an indirect ophthalmoscope combined with scleral depression. The uptake of laser energy is much reduced in areas that have just been dissected and that have been previously detached. Uptake is similarly enhanced in areas of ischaemic flat retina or in the more pigmented fundus. Iatrogenic or spontaneously occurring retinal breaks will best be treated after the introduction of the tamponade agent as the breaks will be flatter and laser uptake more satisfactory. It is unusual for supplementary laser treatment to be needed in the post-operative period.

Internal Tamponade Agents

The choice of internal tamponade agents is between gas and silicone oil.

Retinal breaks in PDR
• Located in close proximity to areas of fibrovascular proliferation
• Usually result in rhegmatogenous element to the TRD

Retinal breaks which are identified per-operatively may be pre-existing or iatrogenic (formed during dissection of fibrovascular membranes). Posterior breaks in flat retina (rare) may simply be treated with retinopexy (endo-laser). Retinal breaks in detached retina require internal tamponade to keep the breaks closed while adhesion is established. If the delamination process is such that there is no residual traction around the breaks then gas internal tamponade should be used provided that patients are able to posture adequately in the post-operative period. Where the membrane dissection has been incomplete (very undesirable) if breaks are multiple, or if the dissection has been complicated by haemorrhage, then silicone oil should be used. Prolonged internal tamponade allows time for the retina to be attached and supplementary laser retinopexy to be carried out post-operatively if necessary. Early visual and physical rehabilitation after silicone is particularly useful in diabetic patients, as posture may be difficult in these relatively sick patients who may have very much reduced vision in the other eye. If bleeding occurs post-operatively in a silicone filled eye it is confined to the retro-oil space. If extensive, this blood can become organised and promote reparative fibrosis leading to recurrence of TRD.

Silicone oil removal is carried out after 3–4 months. The posterior nature of proliferation in diabetes as opposed to anterior proliferation in PVR means that once the retina is totally reattached the risk of retinal detachment after the removal of silicone oil. Buckles are rarely indicated.

Per-operative Complications

The special complications are:

- Intraocular bleeding
- Iatrogenic retinal breaks
- Clouding of the cornea and lens.

Per-operative Bleeding

The management of per-operative bleeding has already been discussed. It is wise to perform endo-diathermy if bleeding occurs during surgery. Blood left in the vitreous cavity clots in a matter of minutes and becomes difficult to remove with aspiration. These clots are adherent to retina and may need to be excised with the vitreous cutter.

Iatrogenic Breaks

During segmentation and delamination a balance is struck between the need for complete excision of fibrovascular membranes and the risk of causing retinal damage. If iatrogenic breaks are made early in the dissection the surgeon will have converted a tractional retinal detachment into a rhegmatogenous one and the dissection itself becomes more difficult due to progressive mobility and instability of the retina.

Entry Site Breaks

Repeated introduction of intraocular instruments is a feature of complex dissection and entry site breaks are prone to occur. Awkwardly shaped instruments such as intraocular scissors can engage basal gel on insertion. Close inspection of the pre-equatorial retina including the ora serrata adjacent to the sclerotomies is recommended at the end of these complex vitrectomies. Tears or dialyses are treated with retinopexy.

Corneal and Lens Clouding

Prolonged vitrectomy can lead to some clouding of the cornea and lens. Corneal epithelium may need to be removed. The use of balanced salt solution plus may be better at maintaining lens clarity.

Post-operative Complications

Post-operative complications particularly related to surgery of proliferative diabetic retinopathy include:

- Bleeding into the vitreous cavity
- Raised intraocular pressure
- Recurrence of retinal detachment
- Anterior fibrovascular proliferation
- Rubeosis iridis.

Early post-operative haemorrhage is usually minor and clears spontaneously within a few weeks after surgery. Bleeding is usually due to inadequate haemostasis at the time of surgery rather than new vessel proliferation. Vitreous haze may be caused by red blood cells spreading from the retained blood in the residual vitreous gel frill. Late post-operative haemorrhage is uncommon and its source is always difficult to identify. It may be from residual undissected new vessels on the surface of the retina or possibly from sclerotomy sites. These haemorrhages usually clear without the need for further intervention. Blood cells can be an important cause of

Early post-operative rubeosis suggests RRD

high intraocular pressure. If the pressure cannot be successfully managed by medical means, or if haemorrhage does not clear or is recurrent then a vitreous washout should be performed and combined with further endo-laser photocoagulation.

Recurrence of retinal detachment arises from either pre-existing or iatrogenic breaks. If membrane dissection is incomplete, it presents as a combined RRD and TRD. Usually in these circumstances the RRD element is much more obvious. Further surgery is necessary to relieve traction and to seal breaks.

Anterior neovascular proliferation is a rare complication and is characterised by rubeosis and a fibrovascular ingrowth behind the crystalline lens to form a retro-lental membrane. Further vitreous surgery involving removal of the crystalline lens, dissection of vitreous base and pan-retinal photocoagulation is necessary.

Rubeosis iridis if present pre-operatively will regress if PDR is controlled by retinal reattachment and photocoagulation. If rubeosis appears postoperatively then RRD should be suspected.

Results

Vitreous Haemorrhage

Visual improvement can be expected in approximately 80% of patients operated upon for vitreous haemorrhage in whom the macula is attached. In the absence of severe complications the determination of the eventual level of visual acuity relates to the state of the macula.

Traction Macular Detachment

Improved vision following vitrectomy occurs in about 70% of cases but this will depend upon case selection and, in particular, length of time that the macula had been detached prior to surgery.

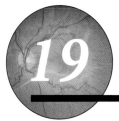

19 Macular Surgery

Macular Surgery
- Macular pucker
- Macular hole
- Submacular surgery

Surgery involving PPV for conditions specifically affecting the macula has developed rapidly in the past few years. It is now well established for treatment of macular pucker and macular hole but much less so for the treatment of either submacular haemorrhage or submacular neovascularisation.

The main indications for macular surgery are:

- Macular pucker
- Macular hole.

Less frequent indications are:

- Evacuation of submacular haemorrhage
- Excision of submacular neovascular membrane.

Macular Pucker

Pathogenesis

Macular pucker is the term used to describe the appearance caused by the formation of epiretinal membrane in the macular area. Tangential traction exerted by this membrane causes the retina to wrinkle and results in visual disturbance. Minor degrees are a common finding in the elderly, are usually asymptomatic and require no treatment. In its simplest form the membrane consists of retinal glial cells proliferating on the surface of the internal limiting membrane. When more extensive and thicker, other cells, for example, fibroblasts and pigment epithelial cells are found. The membranes that form usually remain confined to the macular region but extensive radiating fibro-sheets may form involving a large proportion of the posterior retina.

Symptoms

Clinically significant macular pucker produces the symptoms of metamorphopsia and reduction in visual acuity. Patients describe distortion of straight lines (either horizontal or vertical) and complain that vision is blurred.

Causes of Macular Pucker

The main causes for macular pucker are:

- Idiopathic
- Venous occlusive diseases
- Retinal breaks, retinal detachment and their treatment
- Trauma
- Uveitis

Macular pucker may be mild, non-progressive and need no treatment

Idiopathic macular pucker affects middle-aged patients, and women more frequently than men. Examination reveals reduced visual acuity and the pucker is shown as a wrinkling on the surface of the retina and distortion of surrounding retinal blood vessels (Fig. 19.1). Typically, the vision is reduced to a varying degree (either slightly e.g. 6/9 or profoundly to 6/60 or worse). There is usually a complete posterior vitreous detachment and there is no precipitating ocular disorder.

If PVD is incomplete, remaining attached at the posterior pole, increased traction upon the retina may produce elevation and distortion of the macula (the vitreo-macular traction syndrome). This presents in a similar way to macular pucker and the indications for surgery are the same.

Macular pucker frequently follows venous occlusive diseases particularly retinal vein thrombosis but also may occur in diabetic and other proliferative vasculopathies and retinal vasculitis. Antecedent venous occlusive disease may be relatively minor and the first symptoms noticed by the patient are those related to the macular pucker itself. It is only through the observation of permanent changes in the retinal vasculature (such as collateral circula-tion, sheathing of vessels and capillary drop out) that the underlying aetiology becomes apparent.

Retinal breaks may be associated with macular pucker. In these cases it seems likely that the release of retinal pigment epithelial cells into the vitreous cavity via the break causes a mild form of proliferative vitreo-retinopathy. The macula appears to be a site of predilection for PVR and a patch of discrete epiretinal membrane may only affect central retina while peripheral retina is spared. If the retina is detached macular pucker may be isolated but usually forms part of a more extensive overall PVR picture and this is particularly likely to be found when retinal detachment is longstanding or in those who have had failed surgery. It occasionally occurs as a complication in its own right when retinal reattachment has been achieved by surgery (see Chap. 11) or as a complication of prophylaxis (Chap. 13).

Macular pucker may also follow penetrating injury involving the posterior segment. There is local proliferation around the wound exerting traction on the macula even though the perforating site may be remote from the posterior pole. Other forms of physical injury such as heavy photocoagulation close to the macula may also produce pucker.

Ocular inflammation causing pucker may either be generalised (e.g. vitritis from pars planitis, sarcoidosis or idiopathic posterior uveitis) or focal in the macular region (e.g. toxoplasmosis).

Clinical examination of macular pucker is best performed with non-contact biomicroscopy and indirect ophthalmoscopy is used to exclude peripheral breaks.

Investigations

Fluorescein angiography may highlight an enlarged foveal avascular zone, collateral circulation and distortion of the retinal vasculature confirming an underlying venous occlusive problem or it may show vascular leakage in cases of posterior uveitis. In longstanding macular pucker, leakage from retinal blood vessels in the vicinity of the pucker is more likely and there may also be underlying pigment epithelial damage. In all of these circumstances a more guarded prognosis for surgery should be given.

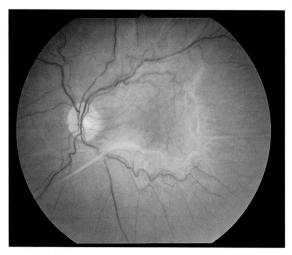

Fig. 19.1. Idiopathic macular pucker. In this case, the epiretinal membrane is quite widespread at the posterior pole.

When macular pucker is present examine the periphery carefully for retinal breaks

Indications for Surgery

Symptoms

The indication for surgery is strongly influenced by the symptoms. If the patient's main complaint is that of reduction in visual acuity, surgical treatment has a good chance of improving this. However, if the predominant symptom is that of distortion patients should be warned that although this may be improved, it may not be completely resolved by surgical treatment. Furthermore, if there is residual metamorphopsia and an improvement in the visual acuity the distortion is sometimes more difficult for the patient to cope with or ignore.

Generally, successful surgery undertaken early whilst patients still have a relatively good visual acuity yields a better visual result. The potential benefit of surgery needs to be balanced against the general risks of surgery and specifically a high risk of subsequent cataract formation and a low risk of retinal detachment. If the vision in the fellow eye is otherwise normal, a reasonable threshold for surgery is a visual acuity of approximately 6/18. If the treatment is successful, the patient can enjoy and maintain binocular vision (Fig. 19.2).

Pre-operative Advice and Post-operative Management

Before surgical treatment is undertaken the patient should be given advice on the prognosis. With successful surgery the symptoms will improve gradually over several weeks. In addition to the usual vitrectomy counselling the patient should be warned that if retinal breaks are present these will be treated and post-operative posturing may be necessary if gas tamponade is used.

Surgical Techniques

The aim of surgery is to remove the epiretinal membrane as completely as possible whilst incurring minimum trauma to the retina. In most cases, there is already a complete PVD and the vitrectomy is simple. Once the removal of vitreous is completed, attention is paid to the removal of the epimacular membrane. The plano contact lens and direct viewing is favoured over the indirect viewing system as the former provides better axial magnification and better stereopsis for the delicate dissection.

Traditionally, an edge of the epiretinal membrane is grasped by forceps and gradually peeled away

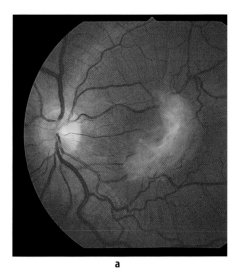
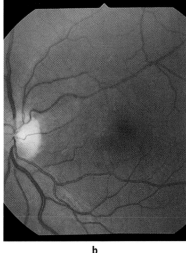

a   b

Fig. 19.2. Macular pucker associated with inflammatory eye disease: **a** pre-operatively; **b** post-operatively.

from the retina, letting go and re-grasping periodically to ensure the membrane does not tear into fine strips. In the absence of an edge picks and needles are used to dissect a plane allowing the forceps to purchase the membrane. Sharp instruments can cause inner retinal damage resulting in petechial haemorrhages on the surface of the retinal and nerve fibre layer.

An alternative technique is to use a back-flush flute needle with a soft-tip cannula and apply gentle passive aspiration over a wide area in the posterior pole. This is carried out with the infusion bottle lowered and with the tip of the cannula closely applied to the surface of the epiretinal membrane. This has the effect of loosening the adhesion between the epimacular membrane and the retina. Slowly, the membrane will separate from the retina over a wide area often extending beyond what could be observed as the full extent of the membrane. It is possible to achieve this separation without using any sharp instruments and employing the forceps only to remove the epiretinal membrane when it is almost entirely detached from the retina.

If retinal breaks are present, care should be taken to ensure that these are surrounded by retinopexy and if any SRF is present around the break, it is necessary to use an air/gas mixture as internal tamponade.

If uveitis is the cause for the epiretinal membrane, then peroperative subconjunctival steroid injections should be given together with an intensive regime of post-operative steroid eye drops.

Results of Surgery

In the treatment of idiopathic macular pucker patients with a mean pre-operative visual acuity of 6/60 improved to a mean final visual acuity of 6/18 when the aspiration delamination technique was used.

Full-thickness macular holes
• Post-menopausal women
• Often asymptomatic
• 10% of fellow eyes affected
• Rapid visual deterioration from Stage II

Macular Hole

Pathogenesis and Classification

Macular hole formation is a relatively common form of macular degeneration, affecting mainly post-menopausal women. Although not fully established the pathogenesis is thought to be that of tangential traction of the vitreous gel on the surface of the macula. The condition is bilateral in 10% of cases.

The classification of macular holes by Gass is used. Stage I macular hole involves foveolar and foveal detachment. Clinically there is a loss of foveal reflex caused by the umbo. Stage Ia is observed as a yellow spot and Stage Ib can be seen as a yellow ring. There may be a slight fall in visual acuity. Symptomatically the patient complains of blurred and variable vision. Stage II is a full-thickness hole. These holes are often eccentric and there is often preservation of good visual acuity. Occasionally an operculum is observed over the macular hole. Histology has shown that this operculum is formed of a glial material with little or no neuro-sensory element. Stage III macular hole is one that is 300 μm in diameter (Fig. 19.3). There is an associated cuff of SRF around the hole. Longstanding cases may also be associated with cystic spaces around the hole. When the vitreous is detached the hole is described as Stage IV. There are often yellow deposits of drusen at the base of the hole. Stage III and Stage IV

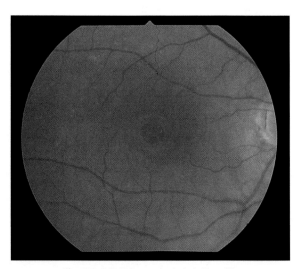

Fig. 19.3. Full-thickness macular hole (Stage III).

macular holes are associated with acuity between 6/24 to 6/60 depending on their chronicity.

Symptoms

The onset of visual deterioration is usually insidious and indeed may be asymptomatic with reduced vision only detected at a routine examination. Symptomatic patients may notice either reduced central vision, a central scotoma or obvious meta-morphopsia with distortion and 'wasting' of objects. Obviously, patients with poor vision in the fellow eye for any reason tend to present with symptoms more readily.

Clinical Examination

Macular holes should be examined with:

- Slit-lamp biomicroscopy using +90 or +60 hand-held lenses
- With eye movements to assess vitreous attachments
- Contact lens for enhanced axial magnification
- Indirect ophthalmoscopy to exclude peripheral pathology.

When a vertical slit-beam of light is shone over the macula, patients with a full-thickness macular hole sometimes report a gap in what they see as a rectangular bar of light (Watzke-Allen sign). If the response is negative, a further proportion of patients may appreciate the gap with the beam shone horizontally. On biomicroscopy using the +90 or +60 hand-held lens the hole at the macula can be seen. The cuff of SRF around a full-thickness macular hole can be subtle. The use of a Goldmann contact lens affords greater axial magnification and allows shallow elevation of the retina to be detected. With eye movements and the slit-lamp focused in front of the retina it is possible to assess the vitreous attachments to the retina. The patient is usually asked to look up and down, then look straight ahead. It is the relative movements of the vitreous to the surface of the retina which give some indication as to whether or not a posterior vitreous detachment is present. The presence of a Weiss ring is the only sure sign of posterior vitreous detach-ment and other observations are difficult to inter-pret and may well be proven wrong at vitrectomy.

The main differential diagnoses of full-thickness macular holes are:

- Pseudo-holes in epimacular membranes
- Cystoid macular oedema
- Foveolar detachments

Primary idiopathic macular holes seldom have well-established epimacular membranes which are identified by retinal striae and distortion of sur-rounding retinal vessels. Pseudo-macular holes are identified by their shape which are often oval and elongated along the direction of the retinal striae. Cystoid macular oedema can be difficult to dis-tinguish from a full-thickness hole particularly as Stage III and IV holes may be associated with sur-rounding cystoid changes. In cystoid macular oedema there is always an 'inner' leaf of the retina present – this may be seen via oblique illumination with a narrow slit-lamp beam of high intensity. Yellow deposits found in the base of macular holes are not found in cystoid macular oedema.

Foveolar detachments are seen as a yellow or white dot. This appearance is caused by altered light reflex from the retinal surface. There is seldom a well-defined circle as seen in a full-thickness macular hole.

Fluorescein angiography may be helpful in that it may show the diffuse petalloid leakage pattern in cystoid macular oedema and a more discreet window defect in full-thickness macular holes.

Optical coherence tomography may be helpful to study changes at the macula (Fig. 19.4).

Rationale for Treatment

It is thought that with tangential traction upon the retina the neuro-sensory elements separate as the hole enlarges and any 'operculum' that is found overlying a full-thickness macular hole is made mainly of glial material with little or no neuro-sensory tissue. Thus, neuro-sensory elements are not destroyed and this may explain the improve-ment in visual acuity that can occur when the macular hole is closed and retinal detachment around it resolved (i.e. the function of the neuro-sensory elements is restored when reapposed to underlying pigment epithelium).

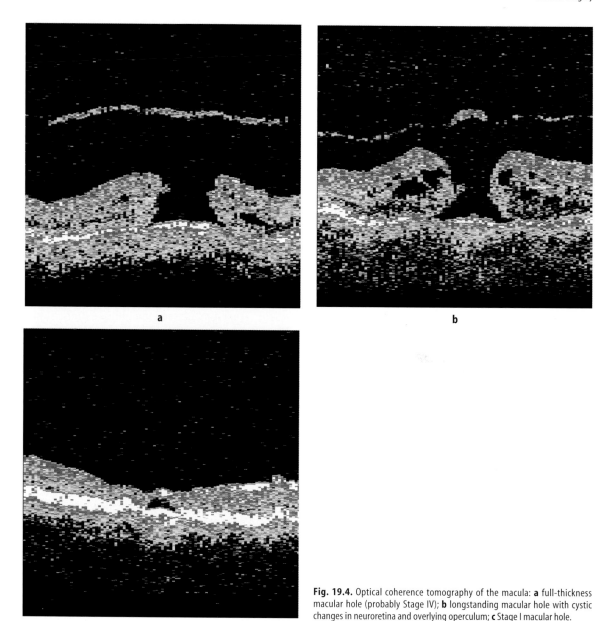

Fig. 19.4. Optical coherence tomography of the macula: **a** full-thickness macular hole (probably Stage IV); **b** longstanding macular hole with cystic changes in neuroretina and overlying operculum; **c** Stage I macular hole.

Indications for Surgery

Stage I macular holes are not treated as the natural history is usually favourable with maintenance of good visual acuity.

Objectives of Surgery

The aim of macular hole surgery is to close the macular hole with resolution of the retinal detachment. The natural history of full-thickness macular hole (Stages II and III) is one of progression with fall of vision over a relatively short period of follow-up (a few weeks or months). Vitrectomy combined with meticulous membrane peel and gas alone may be used to close macular holes successfully. Adjuvant substances (e.g. transforming growth factor or platelet aggregates) may be introduced at the site of the macular hole to promote closure but their role remains controversial as does the additional move of peeling epimacular or internal limiting membrane. This situation will become clearer when the results of randomised controlled trials become available.

Details of Macular Hole Surgery

The elements of macular hole surgery includes:

- Detachment of the vitreous cortex
- Removal of epimacular membrane +/– internal limiting lamina
- Fluid air exchange
- Use of adjuvant
- Injection of long-acting gases
- Post-operative posture.

Detachment of Posterior Vitreous Cortex

Following central vitrectomy, detachment of the posterior vitreous cortex can be achieved with passive aspiration using a flute needle close to the surface of the retina or alternatively, a vitreous cutter near the surface of the disc. By advancing the light pipe very close to the port, it is possible to confirm that vitreous fibres are engaged by the tip of the flute needle or the vitreous cutter. Once engaged, gentle traction will detach the posterior hyaloid from the retina. This manoeuvre may take quite a few minutes and should not be hurried. Even though it is possible to engage the posterior hyaloid quite rapidly developing a substantial PVD can take some time. The observation of a the posterior hyaloid membrane with a Weiss Ring confirms a successful posterior vitreous detachment; this can

> PPV with gas: correct post-operative posture is very important

be extended to the equator if not completely to the posterior border of the vitreous base.

Removal of Epimacular Membrane

After removal of the posterior hyaloid from the surface of the retina, the retinal surface is then inspected for any signs suggestive of epimacular membrane formation. If signs exist that indicate the presence of such membranes (such as retinal striae or minor opacity on the surface of the retina), this tissue should be removed. There is usually a plane between this membrane and the surface of the retina and the removal of the membrane may result at least in partial removal of the internal limiting membrane as well. Fine epimacular membranes are difficult to identify and some surgeons remove the internal limiting membrane to ensure that all epiretinal membranes are removed. When epimacular membrane is fine, the distinction between epimacular membranes and the internal limiting membrane is often extremely difficult to establish. Internal limiting membrane is transparent rather than translucent and has a tendency to scroll.

Fluid Air/Exchange and Injection of Adjuvant

When vitrectomy is complete the vitreous base should be inspected for the presence of any iatrogenic breaks induced by the PVD. These should be treated with retinopexy at this stage. This is followed by air/fluid exchange. There is re-accumulation of fluid at the posterior pole from the vitreous after a few minutes. After a wait of approximately 10 minutes to make sure the macular area is 'dry' adjuvant (if used, e.g. autologous platelet aggregates) is injected over the macular hole and left in situ. Patients are asked to lie supine for 24 hours after surgery with their eyes looking upwards to ensure that the injected platelets do not move away from the macular hole.

Gas Tamponade and Post-operative Posture

Strict post-operative prone posturing and internal tamponade is essential. A 16% C3F8/air mixture or

20% SF6/air mixture may be used and the patients are encouraged to posture for 50 minutes in every hour.

There are many confounding factors influencing the success rate of macular hole surgery. The diligence of posturing is increasingly recognised as being extremely important for the eventual success of the procedure. Patients need help (e.g. physiotherapy to the neck and shoulders can be most useful) and encouragement (from both relatives and nurse practitioner) to relieve the boredom and discomfort of prolonged positioning.

Type of Hole Closure

Post-operatively, macular holes may be difficult to find at all when there is fusion of the retinal edge with the underlying pigment epithelium and total resolution of cystic retinal change and disappearance of SRF. Sometimes retinal re-apposition appears to occur without such fusion and the edge of the retinal break is still seen as an incomplete ring, SRF is absent and improvement of visual acuity may be significant.

Results of Surgery

Closure of the macular hole is usually but not invariably associated with an improvement in visual acuity. This can be expected to give an average improvement of two or more lines on the Snellen chart in at least 60% of patients. In addition, many patients will report disappearance or diminution of their central scotoma and distortion if a prominent pre-operative symptom is much improved by closure of the hole. The removal of distortion is particularly appreciated by patients even in those cases in whom there has been no marked difference in central visual acuity. The visual outcome does not appear to be closely related to the duration of the macular hole (up to 2 years). Indeed, in many patients the precise onset of the occurrence of the macular hole is unknown particularly if vision in the other eye is normal. Those patients with relatively good initial visual acuity (6/24 or better) stand to gain most from successful hole closure as these are the patients who are most likely to suffer further deterioration in their vision as a result of the natural history of the condition.

Post-operative Complications

In addition to the expected complications of any vitrectomy procedure, there are complications which are particularly relevant to macular surgery:

- Early post-operative intraocular pressure rise
- Retinal breaks and retinal detachments
- Pigmentary maculopathy from outer retinal damage
- Visual field defect which may be symptomatic or asymptomatic
- Failure to close hole
- Late reopening of macular holes.

A marked rise in intraocular pressure is frequently observed. This may occur in patients lying supine with a gas-filled eye after macular hole surgery using adjuvant. This rise is usually transient and responds readily to medication.

Retinal tears may be produced as a result of the induced posterior vitreous detachment at the time of surgery. Any small haemorrhage on the retinal surface may signpost such a tear. If undetected they may cause retinal detachment in the post-operative period.

Vigorous dissection of epiretinal membranes or accidental touch of the retina with aspirating cannulae or forceps may cause retinal damage and manifesting as post-operative disturbance of the retinal pigment epithelium.

Visual field defects (usually temporal) following macular hole surgery may occur although the majority of patients are asymptomatic. The way in which these defects occur is uncertain.

Failure to close the breaks is either due to incomplete dissection at the time of surgery or due to inadequate post-operative posturing. In these cases, and provided the patient is fully familiarised with the situation, further surgery repeating the dissection and repeating the tamponade may result in break closure and subsequent improvement of vision.

Late re-opening of macular holes is rare if they have been fully closed by surgery. It may be associated with cystoid macular oedema following cataract surgery.

Prophylaxis

Many patients present with a full-thickness macular hole in one eye and a Stage I macular hole in the fellow eye. However, the natural history of Stage I is relatively benign and prophylactic surgery is not justified.

Special Note

The slightly unpredictable results of surgery, the considerable demands for post-operative posturing in an elderly population, and the inevitable appearance of cataract should ensure that patients for macular hole surgery have to be carefully selected.

Submacular Surgery

The accessibility of the subretinal space to the vitreo-retinal surgeon has enabled exploration of subretinal surgery. At the present time this approach is being evaluated and can, at the moment, only occasionally be advised. It has been used to remove:

- Submacular haemorrhage
- Subretinal neovascular membrane and scar tissue

There is a huge variation in the complexity and the extent of subretinal neovascular membranes. The response to surgery may depend on many factors including the age of the patient, the underlying cause of the neovascular process and the state of the retinal pigment epithelium. There is, however, a role for surgery to play where other modalities of treatment are inappropriate. An example of this is the removal of subretinal haemorrhage.

Subretinal Haemorrhage

Submacular haemorrhage is a sequel of bleeding from subretinal neovascular membrane in age related macular degeneration. The patient presents with a sudden drop in visual acuity. Examination reveals a dark elevated lesion in the posterior pole, the edge of which may have a lighter red colour where the blood is thinner. A large haemorrhage involves the whole posterior pole while a smaller one may be about the area of the disc. There may be intraretinal and subretinal pigment epithelial haemorrhage of varying degree and occasionally subretinal blood can break through into the vitreous cavity resulting in a dense vitreous haemorrhage. Where the bleeding under the macula is not more than a thin layer of blood, these often absorb spontaneously resulting in preservation of some central vision. When the haemorrhage is more extensive, then the natural history is much less favourable. Blood under the retina is thought to be toxic to the photoreceptors and even if the blood is eventually absorbed the central vision is usually profoundly reduced.

Indications for Removal of Subretinal Blood

The indications for removal of subretinal blood in cases of submacular haemorrhage are:

- Fresh subretinal haemorrhage involving the fovea
- Where the haemorrhage is extensive (greater than five disc areas and highly elevated over the macular area)

and the relative contraindications for surgery are:

- Where the layer of blood under the fovea is only a thin film
- Where the area of subretinal haemorrhage is small
- Where the blood is predominantly under the retinal pigment epithelium where it is less amenable to surgical removal.

Subretinal Neovascular Membranes

Pathogenesis

In its most common form subretinal neovascularisation occurs as a result of age-related macular degeneration. Bruch's membrane is breached and new vessels grow and invade the retinal pigment epithelium (Type I). Surgical removal of subretinal membranes in this circumstance invariably leads to the removal of overlying retinal pigment epithelium and the visual results of surgery are poor. In the younger age group the retinal pigment epithelium envelops the subretinal membrane (Type II) and is seen in situations such as the presumed ocular histoplasmosis syndrome. In these cases, response to surgery is more favourable. However, it is also in these cases that the natural history of the condition is usually good.

Indications for Surgical Removal

At the present time surgery is confined to the removal of subfoveal membranes in patients under the age of 50. In these cases, it is judged that photo-coagulation treatment has no part to play and that the natural history if untreated is unfavourable.

Pre-operative Investigation Prior to Submacular Surgery

Fluorescein angiography is performed to determine the extent of haemorrhage and of subretinal neo-vascularisation. The centre of the subretinal membrane is localised as this is useful in the planning of surgery. However, if haemorrhage is large, the neo-vascular complex may be partially obscured by blood.

The patients need to be aware that the visual outcome of these cases is unpredictable.

Surgical Detail

The surgical sequence is:

- PPV and removal of posterior hyaloid

- Small posterior retinotomy adjacent to neo-vascular complex
- Removal of membrane with subretinal forceps.

The retinotomy is made using a small spatula or a 23-gauge needle bent at its tip. The infusion bottle is elevated to encourage haemostasis when the neovascular membrane is grasped and delivered through the retinotomy. The membrane usually has to be loosened gently from its surrounding attachments. If the retinotomy is small it is unnecessary to perform fluid/air exchange or to apply retino-pexy. Both may be necessary if the retinotomy is exceptionally large.

When the surgery is primarily to remove sub-macular haemorrhage the approach is similar. Even if blood clots are present they can usually be delivered quite easily through a small retinotomy and it is not necessary to use lytic agents. When blood has been removed it is sometimes possible to identify the causative subretinal membrane which can then be removed.

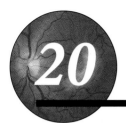

20 Pars Plana Vitrectomy for other Conditions without RRD

- Dislocated lens fragments
- Intraocular foreign bodies
- Posterior perforating injuries
- Uveitis
- Endophthalmitis
- Malignant glaucoma
- Lymphoma
- Amyloidosis

Introduction

Pars plana vitrectomy may be indicated for a wide spectrum of other conditions; the main ones are dislocated lenses, intraocular foreign bodies, the management of posterior penetrating injury, uveitis and endophthalmitis, malignant glaucoma, lymphoma and amyloidosis.

Dislocated Lens Fragments

Previously, the dislocation either of the crystalline lens or of an intraocular lens was likely to have been caused by blunt trauma. However, in recent years dislocation of the lens has become a well-recognised complication of phacoemulsification. This is a rare complication and is more likely to occur during the learning phase of phaco-surgery. The amount of lens material lost into the vitreous may vary considerably from just a few pieces of nucleus or cortex to almost complete loss of the lens.

Management. Minor fragments of lens may be left to absorb spontaneously from the vitreous cavity and do not need surgical treatment. If larger fragments (roughly more than a third of the size of the lens) are lost then surgical removal will usually be necessary. All patients require close follow-up to monitor complications.

Vitreous Surgery

The main indications for vitreous surgery are the complications of:

- Glaucoma
- Uveitis
- Large residual fragments.

Glaucoma often begins with mildly elevated intraocular pressure. Initially, topical hypotensive and anti-inflammatory drops combined with systemic acetazolamide are effective. However, the control often escapes suddenly, and the patient develops high pressure which is unresponsive to maximum medical therapy.

Glaucoma or uveitis may lead to corneal oedema and striate keratopathy and the media further obscured by lens matter in the pupillary area and vitreous. Urgent vitrectomy to remove intraocular lens fragments and clear the vitreous is required.

Small fragments of 'lost' lens material may be left alone

Ultrasound examination can give information on the size and location of the lens fragment (Fig. 20.1). Lenses which have been dislocated for as long as 2–3 weeks show widespread coarse echoes in the vitreous cavity as a result of vitritis. The lens fragments gravitate to the inferior vitreous base and swell rapidly.

The timing of vitreous surgery is controversial. The presence of glaucoma and uveitis indicates urgent surgery (within a few days) whereas in a quiet uncomplicated eye there is no particular urgency and surgery may be delayed for up to 2–3 weeks. However, it is unlikely that very large fragments will be absorbed spontaneously without the advent of complications and we therefore favour removal in these cases.

Removal of Lens Fragments

This can be achieved:

- Bi-manually, using the light pipe and vitreous cutter
- By using heavy liquids to deliver the fragments via a corneal or limbal section
- By use of ultrasound fragmentation in the vitreous cavity.

Lens fragments from the vitreous cavity can be removed by a combination of vitrectomy, the use of heavy liquids, and ultrasound fragmentation.

Excessive manipulation close to the retinal surface is inadvisable. Lens fragments should be lifted by gentle aspiration using the vitreous cutter. Once the lens matter is engaged by the vitreous cutter, the light pipe can then be used to 'force feed' the cutter and mechanically to break up the lens fragments. Relatively large fragments of lens can be removed slowly using this bi-manual technique especially if the lens has had sufficient time to hydrate.

When the nuclear fragment is large, it may be impossible to break it up in this way. Large fragments may require the use of heavy liquid to float them into the anterior segment, and deliver via a limbal or corneal section. Heavy liquid should only be used after posterior vitreous detachment has been induced and vitrectomy performed, otherwise lens remnants can be caught up in the vitreous cortex on its passage upwards towards the pupil and result in retinal breaks.

If an intraocular lens is present surgery is hampered as the exit of the lens via the pupil is prevented. The options are to remove the intraocular lens or to fragment the lens remnant in the vitreous cavity. If the latter method is favoured the posterior hyaloid needs to be detached and removed prior to activation of ultrasound fragmentation. The probes are designed to fragment and not to cut vitreous fibres. Traction from the ultrasound probe on an incompletely detached gel may cause retinal breaks

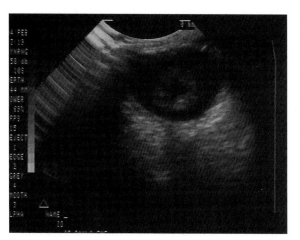 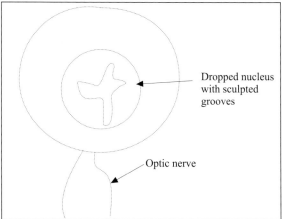

Dropped nucleus with sculpted grooves

Optic nerve

Fig. 20.1. Ultrasound to show dislocated nuclear fragment.

which, if unrecognised will lead to retinal detachment in the post-operative period.

After removal of the lens fragment, a secondary intraocular lens implant can be inserted. Where there is sufficient capsule remaining a sulcus fixated posterior chamber intraocular lens can be used. When anterior chamber lenses are used, peripheral iridectomies are necessary, even though there is no vitreous present as the optic of the intraocular lens can block the pupil, causing iris bombé and angle closure glaucoma. If retained lens fragments have been complicated by uveitis or glaucoma, then it is better to let the eye settle and perform a secondary intraocular lens implantation at a later date.

Advice to Cataract Surgeons when Lens Fragments are Lost During Surgery

The advice given will depend upon the size of the fragment that has been lost. If the fragment is small, then the cataract surgeon may proceed with intraocular lens implantation. However, if the fragment is large, implantation is not advised as this may impair subsequent surgical removal of the lost fragment.

> Aspiration of lens fragments may cause breaks if there is no posterior vitreous detachment

Cataract surgeons should be strongly advised against attempting to retrieve lost fragments from the posterior segment as manipulation of the vitreous via the anterior segment may induce retinal break formation and retinal detachment.

Removal of Dislocated Intraocular Lenses

Removal of dislocated intraocular lenses should be preceded by a vitrectomy. If not, the use of instruments inside an eye with an incomplete vitreous detachment runs the risk of vitreo-retinal traction and retinal break formation. Subsequent to vitrectomy the haptic of the lens can be grasped with intraocular forceps. However, foldable plate-haptic lenses can be quite difficult to grip. Intraocular lenses have to be delivered into the anterior chamber and removed via a corneal or limbal incision. It is necessary to clear the pupil of residual capsular remnants to facilitate this delivery.

Intraocular Foreign Bodies

Pre-operative Investigations

Any patient with a history suggesting the possibility of a metallic intraocular foreign body (e.g. from use of a hammer and chisel) should have a plain X-ray to establish the diagnosis. The radiograph taken with the eye up and eye down, and with the eye looking left and right, gives some indication of the location of the intraocular foreign body in relation to the axis or rotation of the eye. A careful fundoscopy should be carried out to determine the position of the foreign body. If the view of the fundus is obscured by opacities in the media (e.g. vitreous haemorrhage or cataract formation) it is necessary to proceed to further special investigations. Ultrasonography will give valuable information on associated injury, such as suprachoroidal haemorrhage, and vitreous incarceration. When the intraocular foreign body is non radio-opaque, and the fundal view is obscured, it may be detected by ultrasonography. However, this method may be unreliable for small foreign bodies situated immediately behind the lens-iris diaphragm. When the foreign body is metallic a CT scan gives the best information, as to whether the foreign body is within the eye, impacted within the eye wall, or outside the eye. Nuclear magnetic resonance scanning is helpful if it known with certainty that the foreign body is non-ferrous.

Timing of Surgery

All recently sustained intraocular foreign bodies (IOFBs) should be regarded as a potential source of infective endophthalmitis and surgical removal should be effected as soon as possible (within 24 hours). Any patient having a corneal or scleral repair when an IOFB is retained which cannot be removed at the time of surgery should have prophylactic intravitreal antibiotics (vancomycin 2 mg and ceftazidime 2 mg) In some cases perforation may have been as a result of an injury occurring weeks or even months prior to presentation. In these cases there is little urgency to effect removal and surgery may be performed at any convenient time. Some foreign bodies (e.g. glass and aluminium) are non-toxic and may be safely left in eyes which are otherwise stable.

Surgery of Eyes with an IOFB

The objectives of surgery are:

- The prevention of endophthalmitis (recent IOFB)
- The prevention of the toxic effects of the foreign body material (particularly iron and copper)
- The removal of opacities in the media if present (e.g. lens debris and vitreous haemorrhage)
- The prevention of subsequent complications such as retinal detachment by the detection and sealing of any retinal breaks.

Surgery should begin with the closure of the entry site in the cornea or sclera if this has not self-sealed.

> **IOFBs may cause endophthalmitis**
> Early surgery reduces risk

Where the fundal view is good, and a ferrous small magnetic foreign body can be seen to lie in the vitreous cavity, then extraction with a giant magnet is an acceptable approach. If a foreign body is impacted in retina or if the IOFB is non-ferrous, a PPV is necessary. There are a variety of intraocular forceps, which may be employed, to grasp and remove the intraocular foreign body. If the shape and the size of some foreign bodies do not allow their removal by forceps, then a snare with a nylon lasso may be used.

When the foreign body is delivered through the pars plana sclerotomy port, a suitably large sclerotomy needs to be made. (The sclerotomy will be larger than suspected as it is very undesirable to get the forceps with the foreign body stuck in the sclerotomy. This may result in dropping of the foreign body which will have to be recovered again from the posterior retina). The lips of the sclerotomy should be parted, before the forceps or snares are withdrawn. However, it is not necessary to make a large choriodotomy, as the choroid is elastic and will often stretch to allow exit of relatively large intra-ocular foreign bodies. This applies to both magnetic and forcep removal of foreign bodies.

The posterior penetrating wound, impact and any ricochet sites should all be surrounded by endo-laser. These eyes are already primed to develop PVR and cryotherapy should be avoided. Where there are large retinal breaks associated with retina detachment, a fluid/gas or fluid/oil exchange is carried out.

Intravitreal antibiotics should be used routinely as prophylaxis against infective endophthalmitis.

Further posterior segment surgery is sometimes required, to deal with subsequent retinal detachment or macular pucker.

> **The surgical sequence**
>
> - Closure of perforating wound
> - Giant magnet for mid vitreous IOFB
> - Vitrectomy for impacted IOFB
> - Identify and treat retinal impact and ricochet site with endo-laser
> - Use of internal tamponade
> - Prophylactic intravitreal antibiotics

Posterior Penetrating Injury

There is a huge variation in the complexity of cases. This variation is mainly related to the way in which the perforation has been sustained and whether or not there is a retained intraocular foreign body. If not, small self-sealing wounds do not need further surgery particularly if the ocular media is clear so that the fundus can be regularly observed. If a foreign body has been retained within the eye the amount of intraocular damage will depend upon its size and constituency. Large foreign bodies either metallic or non-metallic may cause huge destruction and the prognosis for these cases is bad. Surgery aims to remove as much of the vitreous as possible and particularly the posterior hyaloid which might act as scaffolding for subsequent PVR change within the eye. The timing of surgery takes into account the following:

1. Early surgery is technically difficult – in particular the collapsed globe makes the risk of intraocular haemorrhage more likely.

2. The majority of posterior perforating trauma occurs in young people when there is little chance of pre-existing posterior vitreous detachment. Operating on eyes with completely attached gel is difficult.

3. Delay in surgery carries the risk of intraocular infection.

Surgical Planning

- IOFB removal
- Primary repair
- Secondary vitreous surgery.

As already described, early removal of an intraocular foreign body is necessary to prevent infection and, at this time, complete removal of vitreous may be impossible due to very adherent gel in what is likely to be a relatively young eye.

Surgical planning
• Primary repair (with or without IOFB removal)
• PPV after 2–3 weeks if media are cloudy

In the absence of an IOFB primary repair of the scleral laceration (including the cornea if it is involved) should be performed and should include excision of any exteriorised uveal tissue. The scleral wound is then closed with non-absorbable suture material and prophylactic antibiotic injections into the vitreous cavity carried out. In these cases early vitrectomy is not indicated. It is technically difficult particularly in the presence of a hypotonic globe and the risk of intraocular haemorrhage is high. It is better to wait 1–2 weeks from the time of the perforation to give the gel a chance to detach. If the retina has not detached there will be no afferent pupillary defect and patients will project light accurately. After primary repair the patient should be monitored with serial ultrasonography if the media are opaque. When vitreous detachment is detected, secondary vitreous surgery is advised to remove residual opacity such as vitreous haemorrhage and lens remnant combined with complete removal of the posterior hyaloid. There is little point in further surgery if there is no perception of light. This surgery will generally be carried out approximately two weeks from the time of the scleral repair. Delay beyond this time will allow fibrovascular ingrowth from the perforation site and combined with retinal breaks which may have formed at the time of injury will rapidly produce retinal detachment complicated by severe PVR. If retinal detachment occurs following penetrating injury it will often be complicated by PVR and multiple procedures may be necessary to achieve reattachment.

If the media remain clear following primary scleral repair, the integrity of the posterior segment can be checked regularly with fundoscopy. Under these circumstances, secondary surgery may not be necessary particularly if there is no sign of retinal breaks or of retinal detachment.

Special Note

Sympathetic ophthalmitis remains a rare but occasional complication of posterior penetrating injury.

Uveitis

Vitreo-retinal surgery has an occasional role to play in the investigation and therapy of non-infective intraocular inflammatory disease. Surgical indications are:

- Therapeutic:
  i. Removal of vitreous opacities (haemorrhage or inflammatory debris)
  ii. Removal of epimacular membranes
  iii. Repair of RRD or TRD
- Diagnostic.

Therapeutic

Posterior uveitis is usually managed medically and although in CMV retinitis this may involve intravitreal implantation vitreous surgery has a limited role. It is usually confined to cases of uveitis complicated by vitreous opacity or those in which the inflammatory disease has been complicated by surgical vitreo-retinal disease such as retinal detachment or macular pucker. Vitreous opacities are those which will not clear, either spontaneously or with medical treatment, or in those patients in whom medical treatment has become intolerable, e.g. the side effects from the use of systemic steroids. The incidence of RRD associated with CMV retinitis has markedly reduced since the advent of triple therapy.

Vitreous Opacities

A guarded prognosis should be given when the removal of vitreous opacities is contemplated because of the possibility of co-existing macular disease (e.g. oedema or ischaemia) even if previously unrecognised. Vitrectomy also offers the opportunity to clear the anterior segment of residual opacities (e.g. lens or capsular remnants with posterior synechiae) which will not only help improve vision but will allow visualisation of the posterior pole and help monitor posterior segment disease.

Vitreous haemorrhage is unusual in uveitis and is usually consequent to new vessel formation secondary to the inflammatory process (e.g. in sarcoidosis). Vitreous opacities are more likely to be due to the progressive accumulation of inflammatory debris consequent to the inflammatory process.

Surgical Note

The occurrence of haemorrhage and inflammatory changes in the vitreous cavity often lead to considerable variation in the extent and nature of the posterior vitreous detachment especially as these patients are usually young. Residual vitreo-retinal attachments may be quite firm and removal at surgery may be difficult risking haemorrhage and retinal break formation.

Epimacular Membranes

Epimacular membranes may develop as a result of chronic posterior segment inflammation. These membranes are usually thicker and more adherent than the simple glial membranes of idiopathic macular pucker. Visual results following surgery are more disappointing than the surgery of simple membranes because of coincidental macular disease (e.g. oedema or ischaemia) and there is also a higher incidence of recurrence of the membrane.

Rhegmatogenous Retinal Detachment

RRD occurs in a variety of ways when in association with posterior uveitis (see p. 55). In these cases vitrectomy is usually the chosen method of approach as it is not common for breaks to be sufficiently 'simple' to be treated with conventional buckling procedures. Vitrectomy with removal of vitreous opacities facilitates the detection and localisation of these breaks and will also allow dissection of TRD if it is present. The repair of detachment in these cases is sometimes technically difficult and the prognosis is uncertain.

Diagnostic

Removal of vitreous material may assist in diagnosis. Microbiology, virology, cytology or histopathology are all useful, e.g. to distinguish infective or malignant infiltration from sterile uveitis.

Infective Endophthalmitis

Endophthalmitis may be endogenous or exogenous and the causative agents can be viral, bacterial or fungal.

Exogenous bacterial endophthalmitis

This is usually encountered following cataract surgery, although it may occur following other forms of intraocular surgery. Any patient suspected of an intraocular infection (presenting with pain and accumulation of cells in the anterior chamber and vitreous) should be treated as a surgical emergency. This requires urgent (same day) vitreous biopsy and intravitreal antibiotics.

If treatment is delayed, the infection may result in irreversible damage to the retina with subsequent profound reduction of visual acuity. Subconjunctival and systemic antibiotics are not appropriate means to deal with this condition as the intraocular penetration of antibiotics administered via these routes is insufficient to cope with an established intraocular infection.

The management of infective endophthalmitis following cataract surgery has two imperatives:

- To identify the causative organism
- To deliver antibiotics intraocularly at a sufficient dose to control the infection.

Vitreous Biopsies for Endophthalmitis

Vitreous biopsies should be performed using a vitreous cutter as this obviates against the risk of complications following needle aspiration (vitreous getting caught in a needle and causing retinal breaks). The procedure is performed under local anaesthesia (a sub-Tenon infiltration with 2% lignocaine). A single pars plana sclerotomy can be fashioned temporally and a 20-gauge unprimed vitreous cutter inserted into the anterior vitreous. Up to 0.5 ml of fluid should be removed. Whilst the vitreous sample is being removed, gentle pressure using a squint hook at the equator can maintain intraocular pressure. The tip of the vitrectomy cutter should be visible at all times. When the vitreous sample has been collected the cutter is withdrawn. Intravitreal antibiotics are then injected via the sclerotomy port using a 25-gauge half-inch needle. Our current preference is to use 2 mg of vancomycin and 2 mg of ceftazidime, both of which are constituted to 0.2 ml. The tip of the needle should be observed through the pupil to be in the anterior third of the vitreous. After antibiotic injection the sclerotomy port is closed.

The dosage of other intravitreal antibiotics which are used is: cefuroxime, 2.5 mg; teicoplanin, 1 mg; ciprofloxacin, 0.2 mg; amphotericin, 5–10 µg; benzylpenicillin, 1.2 mg. In the great majority of cases a simple vitreous biopsy and injection of antibiotics is all that is necessary to resolve the infection and over the following weeks and months there is progressive clearance of the vitreous cavity. If treatment has been prompt then usually there will be excellent restoration of central vision. Occasionally, when vitreous debris is unusually extensive a secondary vitrectomy performed some weeks or months later can be performed.

Infective Endogenous Endophthalmitis

This condition is rare and is caused as a result of blood-borne spread by organisms entering the eye via the retinal and uveal blood vessels. It may be:

1. Bacterial
2. Fungal
3. Viral

Bacterial Endophthalmitis

Bacterial infection is most unusual, but in cases of some organisms (e.g. streptococci) may be particularly severe and lead to rapid destruction of the eye. Endogenous bacterial endophthalmitis should be borne in mind when considering a differential diagnosis of an otherwise fit person with unilateral uveitis. The source of the infection must be sought.

Fungal Endophthalmitis

Fungal endophthalmitis is nearly always caused by *Candida albicans*. The main causes of intraocular candidiasis are:

- Direct injection into the blood stream as a result of candida-contaminated lemon juice used as a heroin diluent by intravenous drug users
- As a consequence of the more prolonged candidaemia derived from the tip of an indwelling parenteral line in those whose general condition has demanded the use of the use of these lines (e.g. for post-operative intensive care).

The growth of this commensal organism usually on the tip of the intravenous line is promoted by the administration of large doses of systemic antibiotics enhancing the growth of a usually harmless commensal. Occasionally the cause of candida endophthalmitis cannot be identified.

The eye appears to be particularly vulnerable as other organs are only rarely affected. In drug abusers the patient usually presents with blurring and pain in one or both eyes associated with pronounced vitritis and anterior uveitis. If infection has followed the use of an indwelling line the onset is usually more insidious and the condition more likely to be bilateral. In both situations the clinical picture varies from a few yellow-white infiltrates of the retina (which may lead to profound loss of central vision if occurring at the macula), with relatively little reaction in the vitreous cavity to one involving a severe inflammatory response. In the latter, characteristic puffballs are seen within the vitreous cavity and they are loosely connected by inflammatory strands (giving a string of pearls appearance). Progressive enlargement of a fungal mass from the retina or disc will become adherent to a contracting posterior hyaloid face and result in traction upon the retina causing macular pucker, and traction retinal detachment. The clinical picture is usually typical and the diagnosis established by microscopy and culture of vitreous material (the organism is usually distributed sparsely and may be difficult to find).

Treatment

Intravitreal amphotericin (5–10 μg) may be used in very mild cases of vitritis and systemic anti-fungal agents (flucytosine 10 g per day and fluconazole 200 mg per day for 2 weeks) are also given. When the vitreous is heavily involved or tractional systems on the retina are threatened then PPV is indicated. This will usually be the course to be recommended in young addicts to try to stop macular pucker and TRD from developing but also because of the likelihood of non-attendance of this group of patients. Vitrectomy may be quite difficult in these young patients as PVD will not be well established and there may be close adherence of the posterior hyaloid to foci of infected tissue growing forward from the retina. Haemorrhage is a risk.

Endogenous Viral Infections

Some forms of infection are more likely in the immuno-compromised patient (such as viral inflammation with varicella and cytomegalovirus) but immuno-suppression is not always a prerequisite. The range potential of the infective agents is wide and sometimes the clinical picture can be confusing. Viral infections may affect seemingly perfectly healthy individuals and may present with focal chorioretinitis or as acute retinal necrosis. In these conditions vitreous biopsy to identify a causal agent may aid the medical treatment of these patients.

Malignant Glaucoma

Malignant glaucoma is a rare condition and is diagnosed when raised intraocular pressure is combined with angle closure, a shallow anterior chamber and a patent peripheral iridectomy. This usually occurs after trabeculectomy in phakic and occasionally in pseudophakic eyes. The anterior chamber may deepen using medical treatment including atropine eye drops and systemic acetazolamide. If medical treatment fails, or malignant glaucoma develops again after stopping atropine drops, then vitrectomy is indicated. In phakic eyes, cataract extraction alone will not be effective. The aqueous is thought to be directed posteriorly and the aim of surgical treatment is to remove the anterior vitreous including the anterior hyaloid face. At the time of vitrectomy, a bi-manual technique with deep indentation is used to remove the peripheral anterior gel over the zonules as well as behind the crystalline or intraocular lens. A peripheral iris sweep should be carried out to break down an extensive peripheral anterior synechiae.

Lymphoma

Vitrectomy is useful to establish the diagnosis of lymphoma. The yield from biopsy is often low as the lymphocytes are scanty and prone to autolysis and therefore PPV collecting as much material as possible and spinning down the washings offers the best chance of diagnosis. The vitreous sample should be processed directly in order to maximise the yield. Where there is a discrete patch of choroiditis, an alternative approach is trans-scleral choroidal biopsy though this is rarely performed. In a blind eye, excision might be considered to establish tissue diagnosis which may be helpful for the appropriate treatment of the fellow eye.

Amyloidosis

Ocular amyloidosis is very rare in the UK but a great deal less so in some northern European countries. There is a non-cellular but characteristic veil-like appearance of the vitreous, which may become opaque and need removal by PPV.

Bibliography

Vitreous

Akiba J. Prevalence of posterior vitreous detachment in high myopia. Ophthalmology 1993;100(9):1384–8.

Bishop P. The biochemical structure of mammalian vitreous. Eye 1996;1(6):664–70.

Brod RD, Lightman DA, Packer AJ, Saras HP. Correlation between vitreous pigment granules and retinal breaks in eyes with acute posterior vitreous detachment. Ophthalmology 1991;98(9):1366–9.

Byer NE. Natural history of posterior vitreous detachment with early management as the premier line of defense against retinal detachment. Ophthalmology 1994;101(9):1503–13.

Hamilton AM, Taylor W. Significance of pigment granules in the vitreous. British Journal of Ophthalmology 1972;56(9):700–2.

Hikichi T, Trempe CL. Relationship between floaters, light flashes, or both, and complications of posterior vitreous detachment. American Journal of Ophthalmology 1994;117(5):593–8.

Scott JD. Static and dynamic vitreous traction. Transactions of the Ophthalmological Societies of the United Kingdom 1971;91:175–88.

Scott JE. The chemical morphology of the vitreous. Eye 1992(6):553–5.

Sebag J. Anatomy and pathology of the vitreo–retinal interface. Eye 1992;6(6):541–2.

Yonemoto J, Ideta H, Sasaki K, Tanaka S, Hirose A, Oka C. The age of onset of posterior vitreous detachment. Graefes Archive for Clinical & Experimental Ophthalmology 1994;232(2):67–70.

Retinal Breaks

Davis NM, Natural history of retinal breaks without detachment. Archives of Ophthalmology 1974;92(3):183–94.

Lincoff HA, Gieser R. Finding the retinal hole. Archives of Ophthalmology 1971;85:565–9.

Rosen PH, Wong HC, McLeod D. Indentation microsurgery: internal searching for retinal breaks. Eye 1989;(3):277–81.

Subretinal Fluid

Brown P, Chignell AH. Accidental drainage of subretinal fluid. British Journal of Ophthalmology 1982;66(10):625–6.

Kirkby GR, Chignell AH. Shifting subretinal fluid in rhegmatogenous retinal detachment. British Journal of Ophthalmology 1985;69(9):654–5.

Lincoff HA, Gieser R. Finding the retinal hole. Archives of Ophthalmology 1971;85:565–9.

Marmor MF. Control of subretinal fluid: experimental and clinical studies. Eye 1990–14(2):340–4.

Raymond GL, Lavin MJ, Dodd CL, McLeod D. Suture needle drainage of subretinal fluid. British Journal of Ophthalmology 1993;77(7):428–9.

Asymptomatic Detachments

Brod RD, Flynn HW Jr., Lightman DA. Asymptomatic rhegmatogenous retinal detachments. Archives of Ophthalmology 1995;113(8):1030–2.

Traction Retinal Detachment

Lincoff H, Serag Y, Chang S, Silverman R, Bondok B, el-Aswad M. Tractional elevations of the retina in patients with diabetes. American Journal of Ophthalmology 1992;113(3):235–42.

Ryan SJ. Traction retinal detachment. XLIX Edward Jackson Memorial Lecture American Journal of Ophthalmology 1993;115(1):1–20.

Glaucoma

Schwartz A. Chronic open-angle glaucoma secondary to rhegmatogenous retinal detachment. American Journal of Ophthalmology 1973;75(2):205–11.

Cataract Surgery and Retinal Detachment

Coonan P, Fung WE, Webster RG, Jr., Allen AW, Jr., Abbott RL. The incidence of retinal detachment following extracapsular cataract extraction. A ten-year study. Ophthalmology 1985; 92(8):1096–101.

Cousins S, Boniuk 1, Okun E, Johnston GP, Arribas NP, Escoffery RF, et al. Pseudophakic retinal detachments in the presence of various IOL types. Ophthalmology 1986;93(9):1198–208.

Girard P, Karpouzas I. Pseudophakic retinal detachment: anatomic and visual results. Graefes Archive for Clinical & Experimental Ophthalmology 1995;233(6):324–30.

Greven CM, Sanders RJ, Brown GC, Annesley WH, Sarin LK, Tasman W, et al. Pseudophakic retinal detachments. Anatomic and visual results. Ophthalmology 1992;99(2):257–62.

Javitt JC, Vitale S, Canner JK, Krakauer H, McBean AM, Sommer A. National outcomes of cataract extraction. 1. Retinal detachment after inpatient surgery. Ophthalmology 1991;98(6): 895–902.

McHugh D, Wong D, Chignell A, Leaver P, Cooling R. Pseudophakic retinal detachment. Graefes Archive for Clinical & Experimental Ophthalmology 1991;229(6):521–5.

Tielsch JM, Legro MW, Cassard SD, Schein OD, Javitt JC, Singer AE, et al. Risk factors for retinal detachment after cataract surgery. A population-based case-control study. Ophthalmology 1996;103(10):1537–45.

Yoshida A, Ogasawara H, Jalkh AE, Sanders RJ, McMeel JW, Schepens CL. Retinal detachment after cataract surgery. Predisposing factors. Ophthalmology 1992;99(3):453–9.

Yoshida A, Ogasawara H, Jalkh AE, Sanders RJ, McMeel JW, Schepens CL. Retinal detachment after cataract surgery. Surgical results. Ophthalmology 1992;99(3):460–5.

Choroidal Coloboma

Gopal L, Klnl MM, Badrinath SS, Sharma T. Management of retinal detachment with choroidal coloboma. Ophthalmology 1991;98(11):1622–7.

Giant Tears

Leaver PK. Vitrectomy and fluid/silicone oil exchange for giant retinal tears: 10-year follow-up. German Journal of Ophthalmology 1993;(1):20–3.

McLeod D. Giant retinal tears after central vitrectomy. British Journal of Ophthalmology 1985;69(2):96–8.

Snead MP, Payne SJ, Barton DE, Yates JR, al-lmara L, Pope FM, et al. Stickler syndrome: correlation between vitreoretinal phenotypes and linkage to COL 2A1. Eye 1994;8(6):609–14.

Choroidal and Retinal Detachment

Gottlieb F. Combined choroidal and retinal detachment. Archives of Ophthalmology 1972;88(5):481–6.

Internal Tamponade/Contact Angles

Fawcett IM, Williams RL, Wong D. Contact angles of substances used for internal tamponade in retinal detachment surgery. Graefes Archive for Clinical & Experimental Ophthalmology 1994;232(7):438–44.

Intravitreal Gases

Briggs M, Wong D, Gorenewald C, McGalliard J, Kelly J, Harper J. The effect of anaesthesia on the intraocular volume of the C3F8 gas bubble. Eye 1997;11(Pt 1):47–52.

de Juan EJ, McCuen B, Tiedeman J. Intraocular tamponade and surface tension. Surv Ophthalmol 1985;30(1):47–51.

Lincoff H, Coleman J, Kreissig I, Richard G, Chang S, Wilcox LM. The perfluorocarbon gases in the treatment of retinal detachment. Ophthalmology 1983;90(5):546–51.

Mostafa SM, Wong SH, Snowdon SL, Ansons AM, Kelly JM, McGalliard JN. Nitrous oxide and internal tamponade during vitrectomy. British Journal of Ophthalmology 1991;75(12): 726–8.

Non-drainage Surgery

Chignell AH. Retinal detachment surgery without drainage of subretinal fluid. American Journal of Ophthalmology 1974;77(1):1–5,

Lincoff HA, Baras I, McLean JM. Modification to the custodis procedure for retinal detachment. Archives of Ophthalmology 1965;73:160–3.

Kreissig I, Failer J, Lincoff H, Ferrari F. Results of a temporary balloon buckle in the treatment of 500 retinal detachments and a comparison with pneumatic retinopexy. American Journal of Ophthalmology 1989;107(4):381–9.

Rao P, Wong D, Jones A. Local anaesthesia for vitreoretinal operations: a case controlled study of 200 patients. Eye 1998; in press.

Conventional Buckling with Drainage of Subretinal Fluid

Chignell AH, Fison LG, Davies EW, Hartley RE, Gundry MF. Failure in retinal detachment surgery. British Journal of Ophthalmology 1973;57(8):525–30.

Chisholm IA, McClure E, Foulds WS. Functional recovery of the retina after retinal detachment. Transactions of the Ophthalmological Societies of the United Kingdom 1975;95(1): 167–72.

Gilbert C, MeLeod D. D-ACE surgical sequence for selected bullous retinal detachments. British Journal of Ophthalmology 1985;69(10):733–6.

Lincoff H, Kreissig I. Advantages of radial buckling. American Journal of Ophthalmology 1975;79(6):955–7.

Pearce J, Wong D, McGalliard J, Groenewald C. Does cryotherapy before drainage increase the risk of intraocular haemorrhage and affect outcome? A prospective, randomised, controlled study using a needle drainage technique and sustained ocular compression. Br J Ophthalmol 1997;81(7):563–7.

Smiddy WE, Glaser BM, Michels RG, de Bustros S. Scleral buckle revision to treat recurrent rhegmatogenous retinal detachment. Ophthalmic Surgery 1990;21(10):716–20.

Stanford MR, Chignell AH. Surgical treatment of superior bullous rhegmatogenous retinal detachments. British Journal of Ophthalmology 1985;69(10):729–32.

Wong D, Chignell AH, Inglesby DV, Little BC, Franks W. The treatment of bullous rhegmatogenous retinal detachment. Graefes Archive for Clinical & Experimental Ophthalmology 1992;230(3):218–20.

Retinal Recovery After Detachment

Chisholm IA, McClure E, Foulds WS. Functional recovery of the retina after retinal detachment. Transactions of the Ophthalmological Societies of the United Kingdom 1975;95(1):167–72,

Jay B. The functional cure of retinal detachments. Transactions of the Ophthalmological Societies of the United Kingdom 1965;85:101–10.

Cryotherapy

Jaccoma EH, Conway BP, Campochiaro PA. Cryotherapy causes extensive breakdown of the blood–retinal barrier. A comparison with argon laser photocoagulation. Archives of Ophthalmology 1985;103(11):1728–30.

Complications After Conventional Retinal Detachment Surgery

Fison PN, Chignell AH. Diplopia after retinal detachment surgery. British Journal of Ophthalmology 1987;71(7):521–5.

Goel R, Crewdson J, Chignell AH. Astigmatism following retinal detachment surgery. British Journal of Ophthalmology 1983;67(5):327–9.

Lee J, Page B, Lipton J. Treatment of strabismus after retinal detachment surgery with botullnum neurotoxin A. Eye 1991;5(4):451–5.

Sabates NR, Sabates FN, Sabates R, Lee KY, Ziemianski MC. Macular changes after retinal detachment surgery. American Journal of Ophthalmology 1989;108(1):22–9.

Scott AB. Botulinum treatment of strabismus following retinal detachment surgery. Archives of Ophthalmology 1990;108(4):509–10.

Smiddy WE, Loupe D, Michels RG, Enger C, Glaser BM, debustros S. Extraocular muscle imbalance after scleral buckling surgery. Ophthalmology 1989;96(10):1485–9.

Retinal Degenerations

Aaberg TM, Stevens TR. Snail track degeneration of the retina. American Journal of Ophthalmology 1972;73(3):370–6.

Byer NE. Cystic retinal tufts and their relationship to retinal detachment. Archives of Ophthalmology 1981;99(10):1788–90.

Byer NE. Long-term natural history of lattice degeneration of the retina. Ophthalmology 1989;96(9):1396–401.

Celorio JM, Pruett RC. Prevalence of lattice degeneration and its relation to axial length in severe myopia. American Journal of Ophthalmology 1991;111:20–4.

Folk JC, Arrindell EL, Klugman MR. The fellow eye of patients with phakic lattice retinal detachment. Ophthalmology 1989; 96(1):72–9.

Straatsma BR, Zeegen PD, Foos RY, Feman SS, Shabo AL. Lattice degeneration of the retina. XXX Edward Jackson Memorial Lecture. American Journal of Ophthalmology 1974;77(5): 619–49.

Pars Plana Vitrectomy for Simple Retinal Detachment

Gartry DS, Chignell AH, Franks WA, Wong D. Pars plana vitrectomy for the treatment of rhegmatogenous retinal detachment uncomplicated by advanced proliferative vitreoretinopathy. British Journal of Ophthalmology 1993;77(4):199–203.

Heimann H, Bornfeld N, Friedrichs W, Helbig H, Kellner U, Korra A, et al. Primary vitrectomy without scleral buckling for rhegmatogenous retinal detachment. Graefes Archive for Clinical & Experimental Ophthalmology 1996;234(9):561–8.

Liggett PE, Gauderman WJ, Moreira CM, Barlow W, Green RL, Ryan SJ. Pars plana vitrectomy for acute retinal detachment in penetrating ocular injuries. Archives of Ophthalmology 1990;108(12):1724–8.

Choroidal Haemorrhage

Piper JG, Han DP, Abrams GW, Mieler WF. Perioperative choroidal hemorrhage at pars plana vitrectomy. A case-control study. Ophthalmology 1993;100(5):699–704.

Reynolds MG, Haimovici R, Flynn HW, Jr., DiBemardo C, Byme SF, Feuer W. Suprachoroidal hemorrhage. Clinical features and results of secondary surgical management. Ophthalmology 1993;100(4):460–5.

Proliferative Vitreoretinopathy

Aaberg TM. Management of anterior and posterior proliferative vitreoretinopathy. XLV Edward Jackson memorial lecture. [Review] [50 refs]. American Journal of Ophthalmology 1988;106(5):519–32.

Bonnet M. The development of severe proliferative vitreoretinopathy after retinal detachment surgery. Grade B: a determining risk factor. Graefes Archive for Clinical & Experimental Ophthalmology 1988;226(3):201–5.

Bonnet M, Fleury J, Guenoun S, Yaniali A, Dumas C, Hajjar C. Cryopexy in primary rhegmatogenous retinal detachment: a risk factor for postoperative proliferative vitreoretinopathy. Graefes Archive for Clinical & Experimental Ophthalmology 1996;234(12):739–43.

Campochiaro PA. The Silicone Study. A small piece of the PVR puzzle is put into place. Archives of Ophthalmology 1997; 115(3):407–8.

Cardillo JA, Stout JT, Labree L, Azen SP, Omphroy L, Cui JZ, Kimura H, Hinton DR, Ryan SJ. Post-traumatic proliferative vitreoretinopathy. Ophthalmology 1997;104:1166–73.

Chang S, Ozmert E, Zimmerinan NJ. Intraoperative perfluorocarbon liquids in the management of proliferative vitreoretinopathy. American Journal of Ophthalmology 1988;106(6): 668–74.

Charteris DG. Proliferative vitreoretinopathy: pathobiology, surgical management, and adjunctive treatment. [Review]. British Journal of Ophthalmology 1995;79(10):953–60.

Elner SG, Elner VM, Diaz–Rohena R, Freeman RM, Tolentino FI, Albert DM. Anterior proliferative vitreoretinopathy. Clinicopathologic, light microscopic, and ultrastructural findings. Ophthalmology 1988;95(10):1349–57.

Grierson 1, Mazure A, Hogg P, Hiscott P, Sheridan C, Wong D. Non-vascular vitreoretinopathy: the cells and the cellular basis of contraction. Eye 1996;10(6):671–84.

Hanneken AM, Michels RG. Vitrectomy and scleral buckling methods for proliferative vitreoretinopathy. Ophthalmology 1988;95(7):865–9.

Hiscott PS, Grierson I, McLeod D. Natural history of fibrocellular epiretinal membranes: a quantitative, autoradiographic, and immunohistochemical study. British Journal of Ophthalmology 1985;69(11):810–23.

Hiscott P, Larkin G, Robey HL, Orr G, Grierson I. Thrombospondin as a component of the extracellular matrix of epiretinal membranes: comparisons with cellular fibronectin. Eye 1992;6(6):566–9.

Leaver PK. The treatment of vitreoretinal scar tissue. Eye 1994;8(2):210–6,

Lewis H, Burke JM, Abrams GW, Aaberg TM. Perisilicone proliferation after vitrectomy for proliferative vitreoretinopathy. Ophthalmology 1988;95(5):583–91.

Lewis H, Aaberg TM. Anterior proliferative vitreoretinopathy. American Journal of Ophthalmology 1988;105(3):277–84.

Lewis H, Aaberg TM, Abrams GW, McDonald HR, Williams GA, Micler WF. Subretinal membranes in proliferative vitreoretinopathy. Ophthalmology 1989;96(9):1403–14.

Lewis H, Aaberg TM, Abrams GW. Causes of failure after initial vitreoretinal surgery for severe proliferative retinopathy. American Journal Ophthalmology 1991;111:815.

Limb GA, Little BC, Meager A, Ogilvie JA, Wolstencroft RA, Franks WA, et al. Cytokines in proliferative vitreoretinopathy. Eye 1991;5(6):686–93.

Limb GA, Franks WA, Munasinghe KR, Chignell AH, Dumonde DC. Proliferative vitreoretinopathy: an examination of the involvement of lymphocytes, adhesion molecules and HLA-DR antigens. Graefes Archive for Clinical & Experimental Ophthalmology 1993;231(6):331–6.

Limb GA, Alam A, Earley O, Green W, Chignell AH, Dumonde DC. Distribution of cytokine proteins within epiretinal membranes in proliferative vitreoretinopathy. Current Eye Research 1994;13(11):791–8.

Limb GA, Earley O, Jones SE, LeRoy F, Chignell AH, Dumonde DC. Expression of MRNA coding for TNF alpha, IL-I beta and IL-6 by cells infiltrating retinal membranes. Graefes Archive for Clinical & Experimental Ophthalmology 1994;232(11): 646–51.

Limb GA, Chignell AH, Woon WH, Green W, Cole CJ, Dumonde DC. Evidence of chronic inflammation in retina excised after

relaxing retinotomy for anterior proliferative vitreoretinopathy. Graefes Archive for Clinical & Experimental Ophthalmology 1996;234(4):213–20.

Lopez PF, Grossniklaus HE, Aaberg TM, Sternberg P, Jr., Capone A, Jr., Lambert HM. Pathogenetic mechanisms in anterior proliferative vitreoretinopathy. American Journal of Ophthalmology 1992;114(3):257–79.

Lopez R, Chang S. Long-term results of vitrectomy and perfluorocarbon gas for the treatment of severe proliferative vitreoretinopathy. American Journal of Ophthalmology 1992;113(4):424–8.

Machemer R, Aaberg TM, Freeman FB4, lrvine AR, Lean JS, Michels RM. An updated classification of retinal detachment with proliferative vitreoretinopathy. American Journal of Ophthalmology 1991;112(2):159–65.

McCuen BW II, Azen SP, Stem W, Lai MY, Lean JS, Linton KL, et al. Vitrectomy with silicone oil or perfluoropropane gas in eyes with severe proliferative vitreoretinopathy. Silicone Study Report No. 3. Retina 1993;13(4):279–84.

Ryan SJ. The pathophysiology of proliferative vitreoretinopathy and its management. American Journal of Ophthalmology 1985;100(1):188–93.

Silicone Study Group. Report 1. Vitrectomy with silicone oil or sulphahexafluoride gas in eyes with severe proliferative vitreoretinopathy. Archives of Ophthalmology 1992;110:770–80.

Silicone Study Group. Report 2. Vitrectomy with silicone oil or perfluoropropane gas in eyes with severe proliferative vitreoretinopathy. Archives of Ophthalmology 1992;110:780–93

The Silicone Study Group. Report 5. Relaxing retinotomy with silicone oil or longacting gas in eyes with severe proliferative vitreoretinopathy. American Journal of Ophthalmology 1993; 116(5):557–64.

Silicone Study Group. Report 10. Anterior proliferative vitreoretinopathy in the silicone study. Ophthalmology 1996;103(7): 1092–9.

Silicone Oil

Batterbury M, Wong D, Williams R, Bates R. The adherence of silicone oil to standard and heparin-coated PMMA intraocular lenses. Eye 1994;8(5):547–9.

Campochiaro PA. The Silicone Study. A small piece of the PVR puzzle is put into place. Archives of Ophthalmology 1997; 115(3):4 07–8.

Casswell AG, Gregor ZJ. Silicone oil removal. 1. The effect on the complications of silicone oil. British Journal of Ophthalmology 1987;71(12):893–7.

Elliott AJ, Bacon AS, Scott JD. The superior peripheral iridectomy: prevention of pupil block due to silicone oil. Eye 1990;4(l):226–9.

Franks WA, Leaver PK. Removal of silicone oil-rewards and penalties. Eye 1991;5(3):333–7.

Hutton WL, Azen SP, Blumenkranz MS, Lai MY, McCuen BW, Han DP et al. The effects of silicone oil removal. Silicone Study Report 6. Archives of Ophthalmology 1994;112(6):778–85.

Laganowski HC, Leaver PK. Silicone oil in the aphakic eye: the influence of a six o'clock peripheral iridectomy. Eye 1989;3(3):338–48.

Smith RC, Smith GT, Wong D. Refractive changes in silicone filled eyes. Eye 1990;4(l):230–4.

Heavy Liquid

Bourke RD, Simpson RN, Cooling RJ, Sparrow JR. The stability of perfluoro-Noctane during vitreoretinal procedures. Archives of Ophthalmology 1996;114(5):537–44.

Chang S, Ozmert E, Zimmerman NJ. Intraoperative perfluoro-carbon liquids in the management of proliferative vitreo-retinopathy. American Journal of Ophthalmology 1988; 106(6):668–74.

Liu KR, Peyman GA, Chen MS, Chang KB. Use of high-density vitreous substitutes in the removal of posteriorly dislocated lenses or intraocular lenses. Ophthalmic Surgery 1991;22(9): 503–7.

Retinotomy

Federman JL, Eagle RJ. Extensive peripheral retinectomy combined with posterior 360 degrees retinotomy for retinal reattachment in advanced proliferative vitreoretinopathy cases. Ophthalmology. 1990;97(10):1305–20.

Han DP, Lewis MT, Kuhn EM, Abrams GW, Mieler WF, Williams GA, et al. Relaxing retinotomies and retinectomies. Surgical results and predictors of visual outcome. Archives of Ophthalmology 1990;108(5):694–7.

Iverson DA, Ward TG, Blumenkranz MS. Indications and results of relaxing retinotomy. Ophthalmology 1990;97(10):1298–304.

Machemer R, McCuen BW d, de Juan EJ. Relaxing retinotomies and retinectomies. Am J Ophthalmol 1986;102(1):7–12.

McDonald HR, Lewis H, Aaberg TM, Abrams GW. Complications of endodrainage retinotomies created during vitreous surgery for complicated retinal detachment. Ophthalmology 1989. 96(3):358–63.

Wong D, Williams R, German M. Slippage of the retina. Graefes Archives for Clinical & Experimental Ophthalmology. 1998 in press.

Vitrectomy for Diabetes

Anonymous. Early vitrectomy for severe vitreous hemorrhage in diabetic retinopathy. Four-year results of a randomized trial: Diabetic Retinopathy Vitrectomy Study Report 5. Archives of Ophthalmology 1990;108(7):958–64.

Barry PJ, Hiscott PS, Grierson I, Marshall J, McLeod D. Reparative epiretinal fibrosis after diabetic vitrectomy. Transactions of the Ophthalmological Societies of the United Kingdom 1985;104(3):285–96.

Boulton ME, Foreman D, McLeod D. Vascularised vitreo-retinopathy: the role of growth factors. Eye 1996;10(6):691–6.

Early vitrectomy for severe vitreous hemorrhage in diabetic retinopathy. Four-year results of a randomized trial: Diabetic Retinopathy Vitrectomy Study Report 5 [published erratum appears in Archives of Ophthalmology 1990;108(10):1452]. Archives of Ophthalmology 1990;108(7):958–64.

Flynn HW, Jr., Chew EY, Simons BD, Barton FB, Remaley NA, Ferris FL III. Pars plana vitrectomy in the Early Treatment Diabetic Retinopathy Study. ETDRS report number 17. The Early Treatment Diabetic Retinopathy Study Research Group. Ophthalmology. 1992;99(9):1351–7.

Gonvers M. Temporary silicone oil tamponade in the treatment of complicated diabetic retinal detachments. Graefes Archive for Clinical & Experimental Ophthalmology 1990;228(5): 415–22.

Kishi S, Shimizu K. Clinical manifestations of posterior pre-cortical vitreous pocket in proliferative diabetic retinopathy. Ophthalmology 1993;100(2):225–9.

Le Mer Y, Des Beauvais T, Raynaud JF, Ribeaudeau F. Anterior fibrovascular proliferation. A rare complication of vitrectomy for proliferative diabetic retinopathy, Journal Francais d Ophtalmologie 1996;19(5):369–73.

Pearson RV, McLeod D, Gregor ZJ. Removal of silicone oil following diabetic vitrectomy. British Journal of Ophthalmology 1993;77(4):204–7.

Smiddy WE, Feuer W, lrvine WD, Flynn HW, Jr., Blankenship GW. Vitrectomy for complications of proliferative diabetic retinopathy. Functional outcomes. Ophthalmology 1995; 102(11):1688–95.

Williams DF, Williams GA, Hartz A, Mieler WF, Abrams GW, Aaberg TM. Results of vitrectomy for diabetic traction retinal detachments using the en bloc excision technique. Ophthalmology 1989;96(6):752–8.

Macular Pucker

Akiba J, Yoshida A, Trempe CL. Prognostic factors in idiopathic preretinal macular fibrosis. Graefes Archive for Clinical & Experimental Ophthalmology 1991;229(2):101–4.

Cherfan GM, Michels RG, de Bustros S, Enger C, Glaser BM. Nuclear sclerotic cataract after vitrectomy for idiopathic epiretinal membranes causing macular pucker. American Journal of Ophthalmology 1991;111(4):434–8.

Crafoord S, Jemt M, Carlsson JO, Stenkula S, Shanks G. Long-term results of macular pucker surgery. Acta Ophthalmologica Scandinavica 1997;75(1):85–8.

de Bustros S, Thompson JT, Michels RG, Enger C, Rice TA, Glaser BM. Nuclear sclerosis after vitrectomy for idiopathic epiretinal membranes. American Journal of Ophthalmology 1988;105(2): 160–4.

Kanawati C, Wong D, Hiscott P, Sheridan C, McGalliard J. 'En bloc' dissection of epimacular membranes using aspiration delamination. Eye 1996;10(1):47–52.

Michels RG, Gilbert HD. Surgical management of macular pucker after retinal reattachment surgery. American Journal of Ophthalmology 1979;88(5):925–9.

Saran BR, Brucker AJ. Macular epiretinal membrane formation and treated retinal breaks. [Review, 27 refs]. American Journal of Ophthalmology 1995;120(4):480–5.

Macular Holes

Ezra E, Arden GB, Riordan-Eva P, Aylward GW, Gregor ZJ. Visual field loss following vitrectomy for stage 2 and 3 macular holes. British Journal of Ophthalmology 1996;80(6):519–25.

Freeman WR. Vitrectomy surgery for full-thickness macular holes [editorial]. American Journal of Ophthalmology 1993; 116(2):233–5.

Gass JDM. Idiopathic senile macular hole: its early stages and pathogenesis. Archives of Ophthalmology 1988;106:629–36.

Gass JD. Reappraisal of biomicroscopic classification of stages of development of a macular hole [see comments]. American Journal of Ophthalmology 1995;119(6):752–9.

Gaudric A, Paques M, Massin P, Santiago P, Dosquet C. Use of autologous platelet concentrate in macular hole surgery: report of 77 cases. Dev Ophthalmol 1997;29:30–5.

Glaser BM, Michels RG, Kuppermann BD, Sjaarda RN, Pena RA. Transforming growth factor-beta 2 for the treatment of full-thickness macular holes. A prospective randomized study. Ophthalmology 1992;99(7):1162–72,

Hikichi T, Yoshida A, Akiba J, Konno S, Trempe CL. Prognosis of stage 2 macular holes. American Journal of Ophthalmology 1995;119(5):571–5.

Kim JW, Freeman WR, Azen SP, el-Haig W, Klein DJ, Bailey IL. Prospective randomized trial of vitrectomy or observation for stage 2 macular holes. Vitrectomy for Macular Hole Study Group. American Journal of Ophthalmology 1996;121(6):605–14.

Riordan-Eva P, Chignell AH. Full thickness macular breaks in rhegmatogenous retinal detachment with peripheral retinal breaks. British Journal of Ophthalmology 1992;76(6):346–8.

Sjaarda RN, Frank DA, Glaser BM, Thompson JT, Murphy RP. Resolution of an absolute scotoma and improvement of relative scotomata after successful macular hole surgery. American Journal of Ophthalmology 1993;116(2):129–39.

Smiddy Vffi, Gass JD. Masquerades of macular holes. Ophthalmic Surgery 1995;26(1):16–24.

Wendel RT, Patel AC, Kelly NE, Salzano TC, Wells JW, Novack GD. Vitreous surgery for macular holes [see comments]. Ophthalmology 1993;100(11):1671–6.

Removal of Subfoveal Neovascularisation

Berger AS, Conway M, Del Priore LV, Walker RS, Pollack JS, Kaplan HJ.

Submacular surgery for subfoveal choroidal neovascular membranes in patients with presumed ocular histoplasmosis. Archives of Ophthalmology. 1997;115:991–996.

Thomas MA, Kaplan HJ. Surgical removal of subfoveal neovascularization in the presumed ocular histoplasmosis syndrome. American Journal of Ophthalmology 1991;111(1):1–7.

Foreign Bodies

Slusher MM, Sarin LK, Federman JL. Management of intraretinal foreign bodies. Ophthalmology 1982;89(4):369–73.

Dislocated Posterior Chamber Intraocular Lenses

Margherio R, Margherio A, Pendergast S, Williams G, Garretson B, Strong L, et al. Vitrectomy for retained lens fragments after phacoemulsification. Ophthalmology 1997;104(9):1426–32.

Smiddy WE. Dislocated posterior chamber intraocular lens. A new technique of management. Archives of Ophthalmology 1989;107(11):1678–80.

Vilar N, Flynn HW Jr., Smiddy W, Murray T, Davis J, Rubsamen P. Removal of retained lens fragments after phacoemulsification reverses secondary glaucoma and restores acuity. Ophthalmology 1997;104(5):787–91.

Wong D, Briggs M, Hickey-Dwyer M, McGalliard J. Removal of lens fragments from the vitreous cavity. Eye 1997;11(Pt 1):37–42.

Intraocular Inflammation

Barrie T. The place of elective vitrectomy in the management of patients with Candida endophthalmitis. Graefes Archive for Clinical & Experimental Ophthalmology 1987;225(2):107–13.

Chignell AH. Endogenous candida endophthalmitis. Journal of the Royal Society of Medicine 1992;85(12):721–4.

Doft B, Kelsey S, Wisniewski S. Additional procedures after the initial vitrectomy or tap-biopsy in the Endophthalmitis Vitrectomy Study. Ophthalmology 1998;105(4):707–16.

Han DP, Wisniewski SR, Wilson LA, Barza M, Vine AK. Doft BH, et al. Spectrum and susceptibilities of microbiologic isolates in the Endophthalmitis Vitrectomy Study. American Journal of Ophthalmology 1996;122(1):1–17.

Heiligenhaus A, Bomfeld N, Foerster IM, Wessing A. Long-term results of pars plana vitrectomy in the management of complicated uveitis, British Journal of Ophthalmology 1994:78(7):549–54.

Johnson MW, Doft BH, Kelsey SF, Barza M, Wilson LA, Barr CC, et al. The Endophthalmitis Vitrectomy Study. Relationship between clinical presentation and microbiologic spectrum. Ophthalmology 1997;104(2):261–72.

Thompson JT, Parver LM, Enger CL, Mieler WF, Liggett PE. Infectious endophthalmitis after penetrating injuries with retained intraocular foreign bodies. National Eye Trauma System. Ophthalmology 1993;100(10):1468–74.

Index